# LIPPINCOTT'S
# Computed Tomography Review

**Deborah Phlipot-Scroggins, B.Ed., R.T.(R)(CV)(M)**
Radiography Program Clinical Coordinator
University of Texas Medical Branch
Galveston, Texas

**Wilbur Reddinger, B.S., R.T.(R)**
Computed Tomography Coordinator
Lima Technical College
Lima, Ohio ·

**Richard R. Carlton, M.S., R.T.(R)(CV), FAERS**
Chairman of Radiography
Lima Technical College
Lima, Ohio

**Andrew Shappell, B.S., R.T.(R)**
Instructor of Radiography
Lima Technical College
Lima, Ohio

D0609057

**J.B. Lippincott Company**
**Philadelphia**

Acquisitions Editor: Andrew M. Allen
Editorial Assistant: Laura W. Dover
Production Manager: Janet Greenwood
Cover Designer: Tom Jackson
Desktop Compositor: Richard G. Hartley
Printer/Binder: R. R. Donnelly & Sons

Copyright © 1995, J.B. Lippincott Company. All rights reserved. No part of this book may be used or reproduced in any manner whatsoever without written permission except for brief quotations embodied in critical articles and reviews. Printed in the United States of America. For information, write J.B. Lippincott Company, East Washington Square, Philadelphia, Pennsylvania 19106.

0-397-55157-6

6 5 4 3

Any procedure or practice described in this book should be applied by the health-care practitioner under appropriate supervision in accordance with professional standards of care used with regard to the unique circumstances that apply in each practice situation. Care has been taken to confirm the accuracy of information presented and to describe generally accepted practices. However, the authors, editors, and publisher cannot accept any responsibility for errors or omissions or for any consequences from application of the information in this book and make no warranty, express or implied, with respect to the contents of the book.

Every effort has been made to ensure drug selections and dosages are in accordance with current recommendations and practice. Because of ongoing research, changes in government regulations, and the constant flow of information on drug therapy, reactions, and interactions, the reader is cautioned to check the package insert for each drug for indications, dosages, warnings and precautions, particularly if the drug is new or infrequently used.

*to my new son, Zachary Thomas*
Deborah Scroggins


*to Wilbur Sr., Cheryl Reddinger, Bud Natterman,*
*and The Palmerton Hospital*
Wil Reddinger


*to my first grandson, Nathan Foote*
Rick Carlton


*to my brother, Daniel*
Andrew Shappell

*Examinations usually do not give an indication of the capacity for a subject, but unfortunately they are a necessary evil.*

Wilhelm Konrad Röntgen

# ABOUT THE AUTHORS

Deborah Scroggins holds ARRT certification in both Cardiovascular-Interventional Technology and Mammography. She is the co-author of the *Cardiovascular-Interventional Technology Exam Review* and the *Mammography Exam Review* published by J.B. Lippincott. Deb has 14 years experience in Radiography and has taught for 5 years. Deb is currently Clinical Coordinator of the Radiography program at The University of Texas Medical Branch, Galviston, Texas. She also is the Special Procedures Program Director at The University of Texas Medical Branch in Galviston, Texas.

Wil Reddinger is an Instructor of Radiography and Computed Tomography Coordinator at Lima Technical College in Lima, Ohio. He is ARRT certified in radiography, has 12 years experience in radiography and has taught for 5 years. Wil received his radiography certificate from The Allentown Hospital School of Radiologic Technology in Allentown, Pennsylvania and a Bachelor of Science in Radiologic Technology from Bloomsburg University in Bloomsburg, Pennsylvania. Wil is currently pursuing a Masters of Science in Radiologic Technology at Midwestern State University in Witchita Falls, Texas.

Rick Carlton is Chairman and Associate Professor of Radiography at Lima Technical College in Lima, Ohio. He is ARRT certified in radiography and cardiovascular-interventional technology and has taught radiography for 16 years. He has authored numerous journal articles as well as six books in the radiologic sciences, including *Principles of Radiographic Imaging* and *Introduction to Radiography and Patient Care* with Arlene Adler. He is also writing the 5 volume Lippincott examination review series, which includes *Cardiovascular-Interventional Technology Exam Review*, *Mammography Exam Review*, *Radiography Exam Review*, *Computed Tomography Exam Review*, and *Magnetic Resonance Imaging Exam Review*. Rick is the editor of *Seminars in Radiologic Technology* and *Radiologic Science and Education*, the journal of the Association of Educators in Radiological Sciences. He is currently pursuing a doctorate in higher education at the University of Toledo. He is a charter fellow of the Association of Educators in Radiological Sciences.

Andrew Shappell is an Instructor of Radiography and the Sectional Imaging/MR Coordinator at Lima Technical College in Lima, Ohio where he has taught since 1990. He received his Associate degree from Lima Technical College in 1980 and his Bachelors degree from The Ohio State University in 1986. He has been involved in most aspects of radiography, Computed Tomography, and Magnetic Resonance Imaging while working at St. Rita's Medical Center, The Ohio State University Medical Center, and Maxum Health Corporation.

# PREFACE

This Computed Tomography Examination Review is designed to assist persons preparing for the Examination in Computed Tomography of the American Registry of Radiologic Technologists (ARRT) in anticipation of gaining the Registered Technologist (Computed Tomography) credential of R.T.(R)(ARRT). The review is a useful tool in evaluating the validity of knowledge, pinpointing weak areas for further study, and as a guide to appropriate references for in-depth investigation. The content is also appropriate for students who wish to review a particular subject area during academic coursework, as a continuing education or remediation activity for registered technologists, an evaluation guide for planning re-entry study, and as a review of computed tomography for students in radiation oncology, nuclear medicine, and ultrasonography.

The American Registry of Radiologic Technologists does not review, evaluate, or endorse publications. Permission to reproduce ARRT copyrighted materials within this publication should not be construed as an endorsement of the publication by the ARRT. Any implication of ARRT approval of this book violates the policies of the ARRT. We have never served as a member of an ARRT examination committee to review question items, nor have we had any questions accepted for consideration for the examination in radiography. The questions in this book have not to our knowledge been used for any ARRT examination in radiography.

Every attempt has been made to provide questions that require problem-solving skills from the entire radiography curriculum consistent with subject information in the most popular textbooks in current use. Because of the rapid changes that are always occurring in the radiologic sciences, especially radiography, special effort has been made to create questions that will assure students have been exposed to recent advances in the profession. However, the vast majority of the questions are based on the traditional radiography content areas.

Questions 1-450 are categorized according to the ARRT Table of Specifications for the Examination in Computed Tomography. This permits review by specific content areas congruent with the examination. There is also a 150 question simulated examination that can be used as a post-test following the review activities. This examination is also weighted according to the ARRT specifications. Explanations of the correct answers with suggested references for in-depth study are provided in a separate section. Index keywords to locate the information in the references also are provided.

# ACKNOWLEDGMENTS

This was a project that had been in the back of our minds since we first heard of the proposal to develop the examination in computed tomography. We were grateful that Andrew Allen at Lippincott Publishers in Philadelphia saw it as a viable addition to the growing series of Lippincott Exam Reviews in the medical imaging sciences. We thank Andrew for his kindness and support throughout the proposal, writing, and production stages of this project.

We are indebted to our reviewers who provided a meticulous critical review of the entire manuscript. The changes made as a result of their commentary have increased the value of this book immeasurably.

### Deb Phlipot-Scroggins

I would like to acknowledge the practicing CT Technologists everywhere. Your knowledge and dedication to the profession have helped so many patients lives over the years. Also, a special thanks goes to the students, technologists and physicians in the Medical Imaging Department at UTMB Hospital in Galveston.

### Wil Reddinger

I wish to thank my dad and my stepmother Cheryl for all their love and support. Without the "Win one for the Gipper" pep talks I would not have had the motivation and confidence to finish this project.

I owe a very special thanks to Mr. Bud Natterman, Program Director of The Allentown Hospital School of Radiologic Technology, who picked me up every time I fell down.

I wish to thank Dr. James Cole, Bloomsburg University's finest, Chris Keer, who taught me how to scan, and Mr. Peter Kern, President of The Palmerton Hospital. I wish to thank Cindy Brunner, CT Supervisor at the Lehigh Valley Hospital, and Dr. Bohri, Dr. Bhe, Dr. Tey, Dr. Zacher, and Dr. Gouw, the greatest Radiologists in the world. I would also like to thank Regis Kohler, Tammy Barto, Radiography Staff at The Pennsylvania College of Technology, Bill Bannon, Chief Technologist, The Williamsport Hospital, Barbara Beers, Peggy Brown and my retired boss Rose Houseman, The Palmerton Hospital. And finally, thanks to Barb at St. Rita's, Marsha, Natalie, Jodell, and Mary at Lima Memorial, The rest of the Palmerton Hospital Radiology and administration staff, and my great friends, Nelson Alleman, Tom Zalewski, and Carl Dick.

Rick, Dennis, Andy, and Lima Technical College, Thanks a million!

Mom, my thoughts and prayers always.

### Rick Carlton

I wish to thank my family (again) for their understanding through the authoring projects. Without the infinite patience of my wife and fellow radiologic technologist, Lynn, this book would not have been written. My children, Michelle, Kristöfer, Ærik, Edward, and Michael have not only been understanding, but have been my motivation to continue when it seemed impossible to write ten more questions. And of course I can't leave out my first grandchild, to whom this book is dedicated.

Numerous professional friends have made significant contributions to this work. I owe a special thanks to Dennis Spragg, Associate Professor of Radiography, and Wil Reddinger, Instructor of Radiography at Lima Technical College, who not only contributed questions and always constructive criticism, but have made it possible for me to become an author by making sure our program was running smoothly at all times, especially when deadlines were looming. Thanks are due my frequent co-author Deborah Phlipot and Andrew Shappell, my co-authors on this project, for taking the time to review and comment on many of these questions. All of my students throughout the years, who have demonstrated their professionalism as they never hesitated to point out my errors and shortcomings in a positive manner, have made this a better work. Finally, the consistent support of my authoring efforts by Sam Bassitt, our Vice President of Instruction at Lima Technical College, has given me the necessary motivation to complete this project.

### Andrew Shappell

I would like to thankfully acknowledge several people: Bob and Betty Shappell, my parents, for always being supportive in all of my endeavors; Judy Rayburn and Rick Carlton, for being excellent educational leaders in our field; and Dennis Spragg and Jody Ellis, the two technologists who not only helped me survive my first quarter of clinical education, but went on to become excellent educators. These people have been great examples I hope to follow.

# TERMINOLOGY

It is the policy of the ARRT that new terminology and concepts are used on examination questions only after they achieve general usage throughout the profession. This means that at any given time, the ARRT is engaged in the process of preparing to use new information as schools begin to teach and the profession begins to assimilate new changes. It is therefore common that examinees are familiar with new information that is not yet appearing on the examinations.

**Radiation Measurement**
As of the publication of this book, the ARRT had not yet implemented either dose equivalent limits in place of the outdated maximum permissible dose (MPD) or the SI radiation measurement units in place of the old British system units. Because the profession appears to be moving gently toward the new usage, and because the ARRT advised schools to begin teaching effective dose equivalents in 1988, the effective dose equivalent limits are used in some questions in this book, while the old MPDs are used in others. Questions with both old radiation units (roentgen, rad, rem) and new SI units (coulomb/kilogram, gray, sievert) have been used as well. In addition, there are some questions on the conversions between the conventional and SI system units, also in anticipation of this change. Appendix B provides both the important Dose Equivalent Limits and Maximum Permissible Doses.

Official status was given Le Systeme International d'Unites (the SI units) at the Eleventh General Conference on Weights and Measures in 1960. The NCRP recommended the replacement of maximum permissible doses with dose equivalency limits in 1993 in *NCRP Report No.116: Limitation of Exposure to Ionizing Radiation*.

Radiation protection standards as announced in the 1989 *NCRP Report #102: Medical X-Ray, Electron Beam, and Gamma-Ray Protection for Energies Up To 50 MeV (Equipment Design, Performance, and Use)* have been used for the radiation protection questions in this book.

**Anatomy**
The Twelfth International Congress of Anatomists in 1985 adopted substantial alterations of anatomic nomenclature that were subsequently published in the sixth edition of *Nomina Anatomica* in 1989. Although these alterations have very recently begun to appear

in radiologic literature, they were not used in this book as it will probably be some time before either the profession or the ARRT adopts them.

# TABLE OF CONTENTS

*About the Authors* . . . . . . . . . . . . . . . . . . . . . . *vi*
*Preface* . . . . . . . . . . . . . . . . . . . . . . . . *viii*
*Acknowledgments* . . . . . . . . . . . . . . . . . . . . . *x*
*Terminology* . . . . . . . . . . . . . . . . . . . . . . *xii*

**Using this Review to Best Advantage** . . . . . . . . . . . . 1

**Suggested Study Habits** . . . . . . . . . . . . . . . . . . 3

**Learning Skills** . . . . . . . . . . . . . . . . . . . . . 5

**Helpful Hints for Taking**
**National Certification Examinations** . . . . . . . . . . . . 6

**Directions for Answering**
**the Questions in this Book** . . . . . . . . . . . . . . . . . 9

**Patient Care (#1-90)**
    Patient Preparation (#1-12) . . . . . . . . . . . . . . . 11
    Assessment and Monitoring (#13-30) . . . . . . . . . . 14
    IV Procedures (#31-54) . . . . . . . . . . . . . . . . . 17
    Contrast Agents (#55-81) . . . . . . . . . . . . . . . . 22
    Radiation Safety (#82-90) . . . . . . . . . . . . . . . . 28

**Imaging Procedures (#91-315)**
    Head (#91-135) . . . . . . . . . . . . . . . . . . . . . 31
    Neck (#136-144) . . . . . . . . . . . . . . . . . . . . 44
    Spine (#145-177) . . . . . . . . . . . . . . . . . . . . 47
    Chest (#178-222) . . . . . . . . . . . . . . . . . . . . 58
    Abdomen (#223-267) . . . . . . . . . . . . . . . . . . 72
    Pelvis (#268-303) . . . . . . . . . . . . . . . . . . . . 87
    Musculoskeletal (#304-315) . . . . . . . . . . . . . . . 99

**Physics and Instrumentation (#316-450)**
    System Operation & Components (#316 - 342) . . . . . 105
    Image Processing & Display (#343-390) . . . . . . . . 111
    Image Quality (#391-423) . . . . . . . . . . . . . . . 123
    Artifacts (#424-450) . . . . . . . . . . . . . . . . . . 131

**Answers and Explanations** . . . . . . . . . . . . . . . . 139

**Post-Test: (150 Questions)** . . . . . . . . . . . . . . . 195

**Post-Test Answers** . . . . . . . . . . . . . . . . . . . 237

**Appendix A: References** . . . . . . . . . . . . . . . . 255

**Appendix B: Laboratory Values** . . . . . . . . . . . . 258

# Using this Review to Best Advantage

This review is designed to be used as a helpful tool in reminding technologists of content that was learned some time ago, diagnosing weak areas for further study, and adding a strong measure of confidence to those subject areas in which both academic and clinical success already have been proven.

This review is not a substitute for years of study and practice in computed tomography. It is not possible to prepare for a major national certification examination by studying from questions. Instead, it is critical to engage in the careful study of appropriate textbooks in the radiologic sciences specific to computed tomography, such as those listed in the reference appendix.

To use this review to best advantage, it is suggested that study begin 2-3 months prior to the examination. This review can be used to good advantage by answering questions from each content category section as a pre-test to determine which sections need more review, reviewing reference books, trying additional questions from the same content area, and finally using the post-test as a double check or final assessment of progress.

Each question includes the answer, a short explanation, and references for further information. Answers to questions appear at the edge of the page beneath the question and in the answer section with the explanation and reference at the end of the book.

## Explanations and References

Short explanations are located at the end of the book to keep the question pages uncluttered. The explanation is followed by a reference if further review or study is needed. The short phrases are the index words that should be used to locate more information in the index of any text. Several references that have information on the topic are then provided. The full citations for each reference are included in the reference appendix.

## Answers

Answers are located in the Answer sections at the end of the questions withe explanations (page 139). Post test answers begin on page 237.

## Laboratory Values

There is considerable variation in the ranges of laboratory values considered normal by various authorities. The laboratory values appendix provides you with a guide to beginning to study these with a national view. It is recommended that local guidelines take second place to published values from the various standard reference works.

## Studying From References

It is a good strategy to scan your favorite textbook in each major subject area, skimming headers, bold or italicized words, and figure captions. Most authors emphasize important content by using these devices to bring attention to a content area. Figures are expensive to produce and are used only when important ideas need to be explained carefully. Reading the figure captions is a good way to catch all the high points of a particular text. When something is not remembered, either because it has been forgotten or was never taught or learned previously, stop and study the section. If the entire textbook is reviewed in this manner, few of the "nationally recognized" content areas will be overlooked. The references appendix provides common subject areas for which textbooks should be obtained for this approach to preparing for a certification examination.

# Suggested Study Habits

This is an important test in your career. Do not underestimate your need to study for it. A minimum of a two month plan is necessary to prepare properly. A 2 or 3 week study plan is usually insufficient to permit proper coverage of the multiple content areas you must investigate in depth. Beginning more than 6 months before the examination is not advisable because your ability to maintain an effective level of concentration will be exhausted by the time you begin the critical 1-2 months prior to your test date.

Technologists who have been out of school for some time may need an additional period to get back into study habits. It is advisable to establish a written study schedule and adhere to it. Many students find that requiring double study time when a session is missed is the only way to maintain a regular schedule.

It is strongly recommended that every technologist obtain a copy of the content specifications, listing the outline of subjects to be examined. They appear in the *Examinee Handbook for the examination*, (which also includes the application for examination), available from the ARRT at 1255 Northland Drive, St. Paul, Minnesota 55120, phone 612-687-0048. This document subdivides the number of questions in each content category by subject and is the best study guide. Its proper use permits students to concentrate on reviewing information in heavily weighted areas to gain maximum advantage from the probability of the content expected on the examination.

## General Habits

1. A quiet place away from distractions such as music and talking helps with concentration.

2. Group study sessions are valuable but should be limited to 3-4 persons and should not be the only study method.

3. Concentrate on a single topic area at one time (such as procedures-patient care or instrumentation).

4. Areas of difficulty should be noted for further study by reading a different textbook, consulting with an instructor, or attending a review session.

# Learning Skills

Remember that isolated data is difficult to remember. Try to use concepts to remember data instead of just memorizing the data.

When data must be memorized it is often helpful to use acronyms, such as those in the abbreviations and acronyms appendix. You can invent your own acronyms for data as well.

You can only remember so much information. Be selective in what you choose to memorize so that other more important knowledge is not lost in the process.

Students wishing to further improve their study habits may benefit from reading chapter 2 "Developing Thinking Skills" of the J.B. Lippincott book *Nurse's Guide to Successful Test-Taking*, 2nd Edition, by Marian B. Sides and Nancy B. Cailles, 1994.

# Helpful Hints for Taking National Certification Examinations

Take two calculators that are battery (not solar) powered. Include new batteries for both. Work a variety of different types of problems with both calculators to be sure you know how to use the keyboard before you leave for the examination site. Do not take a programmable calculator to the examination as you could be accused of cheating by entering formulas into the memory.

1. Always read every word of all instructions. There may be a slight change from your past experiences that could cause correct answers to be marked wrong.

2. Most questions are written with the distractors (the possible choices that are labeled a, b, c, and d) designed so there is a correct answer, a closely related choice, and two choices that are less likely. Consequently the best method of answering all questions is:

   (a) Read the entire question and all choices before choosing an answer. Although the first choice may appear correct, the fourth choice may turn out to be a better or more comprehensive answer.

   (b) Look for key words that target important information and don't assume information unless it is stated.

   (c) Determine which two choices are the less likely ones and eliminate them first.

   (d) Choose the best answer from the two remaining choices. When you must guess, this process improves the odds of guessing a correct answer from 25% to 50%. If you guess at 20 questions over the entire examination, this produces 10 correct answers instead of only 5. This could be enough to raise your entire examination score by 7 percentile points!

3. Always work all mathematical calculations twice to make sure you didn't press the wrong key by mistake.

4. Do not spend a long period (more than 2-3 minutes) on a single question. You can mark it and return after you have completed the entire examination. It is normal to have numerous questions that require more than 2-3 minutes. Nearly all students will return to re-study particularly difficult questions after all the questions have been attempted once.

5. It is acceptable to skip difficult questions entirely and return to them after completing the entire examination.

6. At question number 50 remember to check the time and see how you are progressing. If you have taken longer than 1 1/2 hours to reach question 50 you must work faster. If this is the case, when you reach number 75 check the time again and if necessary, mark in guesses for all questions on the answer card. Then continue the examination by erasing the guess and entering your answer. In this manner, if time is called while you are working you will have 25% of the questions you did not answer marked correctly just because of your guesses. These extra correct answers could make the difference between passing and failing the examination.

7. After completion the entire examination should be read a second time to search for errors in marking answers.

8. When re-reading the examination remember that the first choice of an answer has the highest probability of being correct. However, if you can determine that you didn't read the question correctly, or if you have obtained more information from answering other questions, don't hesitate to change an answer.

9. Always mark an answer for all questions, even if it is a guess. With 4 distractors, 25% of all guesses will be correct and these add to your total score. For example, if you only knew the answers to 80 of 100 questions and you answered 73 (73%) correctly, there is a possibility that you would not pass the examination. However, if you guessed at all 20 of the questions you did not know, it is highly likely that you would get 5 more questions right, raise your total score to 78%, prob-

ably pass the examination, and become a certified computed tomography technologist.

Technologists may benefit from the excellent discussion on taking tests in chapter 4 "Strategies for Effective Test-Taking" of the J.B. Lippincott book *Nurse's Guide to Successful Test-Taking*, 2nd Edition, by Marian B. Sides and Nancy B. Cailles, 1994.

# Directions for Answering the Questions in this Book

Select the single, best answer for each question from the four possible answers or completions.

### Answers, Explanations, and References

The *Answers and Explanations* section at the end of the book gives the answer again with a short explanation. Each explanation is followed in bold type by the index keywords and references necessary to locate a full discussion of the content in the question. The complete library citation for each reference is listed in the *References* section at the end of the book.

### Post-Test

The post-test is a simulated examination with the same number of questions with the subject content weighted in the same manner as the ARRT examination. A separate answer key permits a quick evaluation of the total score.

# Patient Care (#1-90)

## Patient Preparation (#1-12)

1. Which of the following should be included in the explanation of a specific procedure when obtaining proper patient consent?

   1. the techniques utilized to complete the procedure
   2. the risks and benefits
   3. possible alternatives

   ___ a. 1 & 2 only

   ___ b. 1 & 3 only

   ___ c. 2 & 3 only

   ___ d. 1, 2, & 3

2. Which of the following documents are part of the patient's medical record?

   1. record of medications given
   2. consent forms
   3. radiographs

   ___ a. 1 & 2 only

   ___ b. 1 & 3 only

   ___ c. 2 & 3 only

   ___ d. 1, 2, & 3

3. Which of the following is a valid method of verifying patient identification?

   1. questioning patient
   2. reading wrist identification band
   3. checking bed name plate

   ___ a. 1 only

   ___ b. 2 only

   ___ c. 3 only

   ___ d. 1, 2, & 3

4. What legal doctrine, now in decline, holds that the employer is responsible for the acts of the radiographer?

    __ a. assault and battery

    __ b. res ipsa loquitur

    __ c. respondeat superior

    __ d. habeas corpus

5. In which of the following situations would it be possible to proceed with a radiographic procedure although the patient clearly indicates refusal?

    1. the patient is a minor and the parents give permission

    2. the patient is over age 95

    3. the patient is a prisoner in the custody of an officer of the law, who gives permission

    __ a. 1 & 2 only

    __ b. 1 & 3 only

    __ c. 2 & 3 only

    __ d. 1, 2, & 3

6. What is the appropriate action if a patient indicates pain in the left leg, but a right leg examination is ordered?

    __ a. perform a left leg examination

    __ b. perform a right leg examination

    __ c. perform both a left and right leg examination

    __ d. request clarification from the ordering physician

7. What is the most appropriate action if a patient denies knowledge of the possible effects of the use of contrast material?

    __ a. terminate the examination

    __ b. explain the effects and then proceed

    __ c. proceed with the examination

    __ d. consult with legal counsel

8. When must a patient sign a consent form?

  __ a.  when a contrast agent is used

  __ b.  when the examination time exceeds 30 minutes

  __ c.  if family cannot be present during the examination

  __ d.  if trauma is suspected

9. Which of the following technologists responsibilities must be checked prior to starting a study?

  1.  correct patient position

  2.  proper breathing instructions

  3.  proper selection of technical factors

  __ a.  1 & 2 only

  __ b.  1 & 3 only

  __ c.  2 & 3 only

  __ d.  1, 2 & 3

10. Which of the following will have an effect on patient positioning for a CT exam?

  1.  desired plane of anatomy to be imaged

  2.  ability of the patient to cooperate

  3.  limitation of the gantry angulation

  __ a.  1 & 2 only

  __ b.  1 & 3 only

  __ c.  2 & 3 only

  __ d.  1, 2 & 3

11. What may happen as a result of patient movement during an examination?

  __ a.  loss of diagnostic information

  __ b.  low tissue density

  __ c.  high tissue density

  __ d.  increased window level adjustments

12. Which of the following should be checked prior to giving a patient contrast media?

    1.   allergies
    2.   cardiac history
    3.   renal history

      ___ a.  1 only
      ___ b.  2 only
      ___ c.  3 only
      ___ d.  1, 2, & 3

## Assessment and Monitoring      (#13-30)

13. What is the normal range of diastolic pressure for adults?

      ___ a.  40 - 80 mm Hg
      ___ b.  60 - 80 mm Hg
      ___ c.  90 - 120 mm Hg
      ___ d.  110 - 140 mm Hg

14. What is the average normal range of pulse rates for an infant?

      ___ a.  20 - 40 beats per minute
      ___ b.  50 - 70 beats per minute
      ___ c.  80 - 100 beats per minute
      ___ d.  115 - 130 beats per minute

15. The patient in insulin shock who is still conscious requires which of the following?

      ___ a.  something with sugar
      ___ b.  something salty
      ___ c.  more insulin
      ___ d.  an immediate transfusion

16. Which of the following terms describes a state of oxygen deficiency at the tissue level?

      ___ a.  hypotension
      ___ b.  hypothermia
      ___ c.  hypoxia
      ___ d.  apnea

17. What is another term for fainting?

___ a. palsy

___ b. syncope

___ c. dysphagia

___ d. indoxyluria

18. What is the range of normal respiratory rates for an adult?

___ a. 5 - 8 respirations per minute

___ b. 10 - 20 respirations per minute

___ c. 20 - 30 respirations per minute

___ d. 30 - 40 respirations per minute

19. Which of the following delivers the highest concentration of oxygen to the patient?

___ a. nonrebreathing mask

___ b. aerosol mask

___ c. partial rebreathing mask

___ d. nasal cannula

20. Which of the following conditions would indicate difficulty breathing?

___ a. dysplasia

___ b. dyspnea

___ c. dysphylaxia

___ d. dystaxia

21. What is the correct order for administering basic life support?

___ a. circulation, breathing, airway

___ b. airway, circulation, breathing

___ c. breathing, circulation, airway

___ d. airway, breathing, circulation

22. Which of the following indicates the time frame for CPR to be started on a cardiac arrest victim before there is a risk of brain damage?

    ___ a.  1 - 3 minutes

    ___ b.  4 - 6 minutes

    ___ c.  8 - 10 minutes

    ___ d.  15 minutes

23. What should be your first action if a patient is bleeding profusely from an open wound?

    ___ a.  call for a nurse

    ___ b.  apply direct pressure to the wound

    ___ c.  call for a doctor

    ___ d.  finish the scan as quickly as possible

24. What type of shock is caused by an excessive loss of blood?

    ___ a.  cardiogenic

    ___ b.  septic

    ___ c.  anaphylactic

    ___ d.  hypovolemic

25. Which of the following is a potential problem for a patient scheduled for a mid morning examination who has had a normal dose of insulin the previous night but has been NPO since midnight?

    ___ a.  diabetic coma

    ___ b.  insulin shock

    ___ c.  dehydration

    ___ d.  angina

26. Which of the following describes the drug Nitroglycerin?

    ___ a.  vasoconstrictor

    ___ b.  anesthetic

    ___ c.  analgesic

    ___ d.  vasodilator

27. What is represented by the term PTT as applied to a laboratory value?

   __ a.  prothrombin time

   __ b.  thromboplastin time

   __ c.  partial thromboplastin time

   __ d.  partial prothrombin time

28. Which of the following is considered to be within the normal range for an average adult PTT coagulation study?

   __ a.  20 - 37 seconds

   __ b.  60 - 97 seconds

   __ c.  100 - 150 seconds

   __ d.  5 minutes

29. Which of the following is considered to be within the normal range for an average adult PT coagulation study.

   __ a.  10 - 14 seconds

   __ b.  20 - 24 seconds

   __ c.  30 - 34 seconds

   __ d.  1 minute

30. Which of the following is within the normal range for an average adult BUN?

   __ a.  5 mmol/l

   __ b.  20 mmol/l

   __ c.  100 mmol/l

   __ d.  850 mmol/l

# IV Procedures                                 *(#31-54)*

31. What sterilization method uses subjection to pressurized steam at about 250° F for a period of time?

   __ a.  fractional

   __ b.  dryheat

   __ c.  chemical

   __ d.  autoclaving

32. Enteric precautions are used to prevent infection transmitted by contact with which substance?

___ a. blood

___ b. airborne droplets

___ c. saliva

___ d. fecal material

33. Which of the following describes reducing the probability of infectious organisms being transmitted to someone who is susceptible?

___ a. disinfection

___ b. medical asepsis

___ c. sterilization

___ d. cleanliness

34. What is the proper action to take when sterilization of an object is in question?

___ a. resterilize the object for 50% of original sterilization time

___ b. disinfect the object

___ c. discard the object

___ d. if someone else believes the object is sterile, it may be used

35. Which of the following describes the first stage of an infection?

___ a. prodromal phase

___ b. full phase

___ c. incubation period

___ d. convalescent phase

36. Which of the following are most resistant to aseptic technique?

___ a. yeasts

___ b. streptococci bacteria

___ c. bacillic spore bacteria

___ d. moving protozoa

37. What term describes the destruction of pathogens by using chemicals?

    ___ a. disinfection

    ___ b. medical asepsis

    ___ c. sterilization

    ___ d. cleanliness

38. Which method of sterilization is the most effective and convenient for items that can withstand high temperatures?

    ___ a. gas

    ___ b. steam

    ___ c. chemicals

    ___ d. dry heat

39. What is a nosocomial infection?

    ___ a. an infection acquired by a patient while in a health-care institution

    ___ b. an infection of the upper nasal passages

    ___ c. an infection of the inferior nasal conchae

    ___ d. an virulent microorganism that resists sterilization

40. Which of the following is the most common butterfly needle gauge used in the diagnostic imaging department?

    ___ a. 16-gauge

    ___ b. 19-gauge

    ___ c. 25-gauge

    ___ d. 27-gauge

41. Which of the following includes a parenteral drug route?

    1. intramuscular
    2. intravenous
    3. oral

    ___ a. 1 & 2 only

    ___ b. 1 & 3 only

    ___ c. 2 & 3 only

    ___ d. 1, 2, & 3

42. How long must a patient be observed following the administration of a medication?

___ a. 5 minutes

___ b. 10 minutes

___ c. 30 minutes

___ d. 1 hour

43. Which of the following describes a plastic tubing with a needle through the tubing for insertion into a vein?

___ a. angiocatheter

___ b. "piggypack"

___ c. tuberculin syringe

___ d. butterfly needle

44. Which of the following locations is preferred for the introduction of IV contrast media?

___ a. cephalic vein

___ b. antecubital vein

___ c. lateral vein

___ d. subclavian vein

45. Which of the following terms indicates an injection made between the layers of the skin?

___ a. subcutaneous

___ b. intramuscular

___ c. intradermal

___ d. intravenous

46. Which vein should be used for an IV infusion that requires less than 1 hour for administration?

___ a. cephalic vein

___ b. antecubital vein

___ c. lateral vein

___ d. subclavian vein

47. Which of the following veins should be used for a prolonged IV infusion?

1. forearm veins
2. back of the hand veins
3. antecubital vein

___ a. 1 & 2 only
___ b. 1 & 3 only
___ c. 2 & 3 only
___ d. 1, 2, & 3

48. Which of the following would indicate selecting a large vein in the forearm for administering a solution?

1. introduction of a hypertonic solution
2. a solution to be administered rapidly
3. a viscid solution

___ a. 1 & 2 only
___ b. 1 & 3 only
___ c. 2 & 3 only
___ d. 1, 2, & 3

49. Which of the following amounts of contrast media would be used for a single scan sequence?

___ a. 20 - 50 ml
___ b. 60 - 90 ml
___ c. 100 - 180 ml
___ d. 200 - 300 ml

50. Which of the following would be the proper delay between initiating injection and scanning of the chest?

___ a. 10 - 20 sec.
___ b. 30 - 45 sec.
___ c. 1 min.
___ d. 2 min.

51. Which of the following would be the proper delay between initiating injection and scanning of the liver?

    ___ a. 10 - 20 sec.

    ___ b. 30 - 45 sec.

    ___ c. 2 min.

    ___ d. 3 min.

52. Why is it necessary to delay scanning of the liver after the injection of contrast media?

    ___ a. allow time for contrast to reach the splenic artery

    ___ b. allow time for contrast to reach the portal vein

    ___ c. allow time for contrast to reach the hepatic artery

    ___ d. allow time for contrast to reach the celiac artery

53. What is the patient preparation for a brain scan without using contrast media?

    ___ a. no preparation

    ___ b. nothing orally for 4 hours before the examination

    ___ c. nothing orally after midnight

    ___ d. IV heparin 1 hour before exam

54. Which of the following would be the proper delay between initiating injection and scanning of the pancreas?

    ___ a. 5 - 10 sec.

    ___ b. 20 - 30 sec.

    ___ c. 2 min.

    ___ d. 3 min.

# Contrast Agents                                    (#55-81)

55. Which of the following is a disadvantage associated with using a contrast media with a high iodine concentration?

    ___ a. decreased persistence

    ___ b. decreased vessel opacity

    ___ c. increased contrast media viscosity

    ___ d. decreased concentration

56. Which of the following pre-procedural preparations can be done to prevent possible renal failure following an ionic contrast injection?

    __ a. dehydration

    __ b. heparinization

    __ c. hydration

    __ d. sedation

57. Which of the following are true statements concerning ionic contrast media?

    1. ionic medias dissociates into two charged particles for every three iodine molecules present

    2. ionic medias are hyperosmolar solutions

    3. ionic medias are not water soluble

        __ a. 1 & 2 only

        __ b. 1 & 3 only

        __ c. 2 & 3 only

        __ d. 1, 2, & 3

58. What causes positive contrast material to produce an area of reduced image density?

    __ a. scatter of primary photons

    __ b. absorption of primary photons

    __ c. scatter of secondary photons

    __ d. absorption of secondary photons

59. Which of the following are possible adverse side effects of contrast media injections?

    1. headaches

    2. aphasia

    3. unconsciousness

        __ a. 1 & 2 only

        __ b. 1 & 3 only

        __ c. 2 & 3 only

        __ d. 1, 2, & 3

60. Which of the following medications would relax vascular walls to permit greater blood flow?

    ___ a.  stimulant

    ___ b.  diuretic

    ___ c.  vasodilator

    ___ d.  anticoagulant

61. Which is used for visualization of the gastrointestinal tract when a perforation is **NOT** suspected?

    ___ a.  barium sulfite

    ___ b.  barium sulfate

    ___ c.  potassium sulfite

    ___ d.  potassium sulfate

62. Which of the following is not an acceptable method of cleansing the bowel before placing barium in the rectum?

    ___ a.  castor oil

    ___ b.  bismuth laxative

    ___ c.  saline enema

    ___ d.  soap suds enema

63. When scanning for a pelvic malignancy, how much rectal contrast should be used?

    ___ a.  50 - 75 ml

    ___ b.  100 - 150 ml

    ___ c.  300 - 500 ml

    ___ d.  500 - 1000 ml

64. Which of the following decreases the viscosity of contrast media?

    ___ a.  cooling

    ___ b.  warming

    ___ c.  maintaining at a constant temperature

    ___ d.  decreasing pressure

65. Which of the following are true regarding excessive release of histamine in the body?

   1. bronchial and tracheal smooth muscle is constricted
   2. induces capillary dilation
   3. lowers blood pressure

   __ a.  1 & 2
   __ b.  1 & 3
   __ c.  2 & 3
   __ d.  1, 2, & 3

66. What can be done if a patient is unable to ingest oral contrast?

   __ a.  the exam is terminated
   __ b.  the contrast is given through the rectum
   __ c.  the contrast can be injected through a nasogastric tube
   __ d.  the contrast is given by a drip infusion

67. What does it mean to administer drugs parenterally?

   __ a.  IV or by injection
   __ b.  orally
   __ c.  rectally
   __ d.  via a nasal gastric tube

68. For a patient receiving an IV solution, how high above the vein should the bag of solution be kept?

   __ a.  10 - 12 inches
   __ b.  18 - 20 inches
   __ c.  25 - 30 inches
   __ d.  35 - 40 inches

69. What is the usual rate of flow for an adult with an IV in use?

   __ a.  2 - 4 drops per minute
   __ b.  15 - 20 drops per minute
   __ c.  60 - 75 drops per minute
   __ d.  100 - 125 drops per minute

70. Gastrografin and Gastroview, are examples of what type of contrast media?

___ a. intravenous contrast

___ b. drip infusion contrast

___ c. intrathecal contrast

___ d. oral contrast

71. Which of the following mixtures would yield an acceptable concentration of oral contrast media that is optimal for CT scanning of the abdomen?

___ a. 3ml of 60% oral contrast solution to 100ml of water

___ b. 30ml of 60% oral contrast solution to 100ml of water

___ c. 50ml of 60% oral contrast solution to 100ml of water

___ d. 100 ml of 60% oral contrast solution to 100ml of water

72. What is the total amount of oral contrast material that should be given when scanning the adult upper abdomen?

___ a. 25 - 50 ml

___ b. 100 - 200 ml

___ c. 300 - 1,000 ml

___ d. 2,000 plus ml

73. Which of the following is an appropriate enema when preparing a patient for a pelvic scan?

___ a. 50 - 100 ml

___ b. 150 - 250 ml

___ c. 300 - 1000 ml

___ d. 2000 - 3000 ml

74. What is the purpose for using a tampon during pelvic scanning?

   1. produces an entrapment of air
   2. aid in anatomical localization
   3. demonstrates the vagina

   ___ a.  1 & 2 only

   ___ b.  1 & 3 only

   ___ c.  2 & 3 only

   ___ d.  1, 2, & 3

75. Which of the following may cause beam hardening artifacts when giving a barium sulfate suspension?

   1. suspension of too low a concentration
   2. suspension of too high a concentration
   3. delays of scanning after ingestion
   4. scanning starting minutes after ingestion

   ___ a.  1 & 2 only

   ___ b.  1 & 3 only

   ___ c.  2 & 3 only

   ___ d.  1, 2, & 3

76. What is the purpose of the heating device on an automatic pressure injector?

   ___ a.  decrease contrast media flow rate

   ___ b.  decrease contrast media viscosity

   ___ c.  decrease  friction of the internal parts of the injector

   ___ d.  increase the plunger velocity

77. Which of the following increases the delivery rate of contrast material when a constant pressure injector is used?

   ___ a.  increased contrast viscosity

   ___ b.  increased catheter length

   ___ c.  increased catheter diameter

   ___ d.  increased contrast concentration

78. Which type of contrast media studies should be performed first?

    ___ a. iodine

    ___ b. barium

    ___ c. iodinated oil

    ___ d. air

79. Which of the following would be an appropriate amount of contrast material to drink prior to a study of the stomach?

    ___ a. 10 - 50 ml

    ___ b. 100 - 200 ml

    ___ c. 350 - 500 ml

    ___ d. 500 - 1000 ml

80. For an exam of the liver which of the following contrast material injections rates might be used?

    ___ a. 10 - 50 ml, in one minute

    ___ b. 150 - 180 ml, in two minutes

    ___ c. 250 - 300 ml, in two minutes

    ___ d. 500 - 1000 ml, in four minutes

81. How long is the injection time for 30 ml of contrast media delivered at 3.7 ml/sec?

    ___ a. 0.1 sec

    ___ b. 4.5 sec

    ___ c. 8.1 sec

    ___ d. 111 sec

# Radiation Safety                                          (#82-90)

82. Most early scanners employed which of the following single kVp selections?

    ___ a. between 80 and 90 kVp

    ___ b. between 100 and 110 kVp

    ___ c. between 120 and 130 kVp

    ___ d. between 140 and 150 kVp

83. Which of the following physical interactions between radiation and matter result in the production of the most scatter radiation from which occupational exposure occurs?

___ a.  photoelectric effect

___ b.  Compton effect

___ c.  pair production

___ d.  coherent scatter

84. Which of the following indicates the maximum rate of x-ray output?

___ a.  tube-detector system

___ b.  kVp

___ c.  scan time

___ d.  mA

85. Which of the following would contribute to higher patient doses during a CT scan?

1.  multiple scans at a single level
2.  low mAs settings
3.  high-resolution scans with long scan times

___ a.  1 & 2 only

___ b.  1 & 3 only

___ c.  2 & 3 only

___ d.  1, 2, & 3

86. Which of the following is a typical skin dose using the manufacturer's recommended mAs and kVp settings when doing a scanogram?

___ a.  0.005 - .05 rad

___ b.  0.05 - 0.1 rad

___ c.  1 - 2 rads

___ d.  2 - 4 rads

87. Which of the following is true regarding the reduced effectiveness of shielding a patient during a CT scan?

1. lead from shields causes artifacts on the image
2. low level scatter radiation is increased
3. rotational scheme of the x-ray source reduces shield effectiveness

___ a. 1 & 2 only

___ b. 1 & 3 only

___ c. 2 & 3 only

___ d. 1, 2, & 3

88. Which trimester is the most critical period to avoid irradiation of the embryo or the fetus?

___ a. 1st

___ b. 2nd

___ c. 3rd

___ d. all trimesters are equally critical

89. What is the MPD for a pregnant woman?

___ a. 0.025 rem

___ b. 0.25 rem

___ c. 0.5 rem

___ d. 2.5 rem

90. Which of the following body tissues is the most radiosensitive?

___ a. solid visceral organs

___ b. blood forming organs

___ c. muscular muscles

___ d. central nervous system

# Imaging Procedures  *(#91-315)*

## Head *(#91-135)*

91. What is the most common scout view for a CT of the brain?

    __ a.  lateral

    __ b.  AP

    __ c.  PA

    __ d.  mid sagittal

92. What angle is used for axial sections of a routine brain study?

    __ a.  Parallel to the infraorbitomeatal line

    __ b.  Parallel to the orbitomeatal line

    __ c.  10-20 degrees to the orbitomeatal line

    __ d.  30-40 degrees to the orbitomeatal line

93. What is the most common range for axial section thickness for routine brain exams?

    __ a.  1-3 mm

    __ b.  3-5 mm

    __ c.  5-10 mm

    __ d.  always 3 mm

94. Which of the following may be used as contrast medium for head exams?

    1.  intravenous contrast media
    2.  positive intrathecal contrast media
    3.  oral contrast media

    __ a.  1 and 2

    __ b.  1 and 3

    __ c.  2 and 3

    __ d.  1, 2, & 3

95. What is the usual patient position for a routine head exam?

    — a.  supine, head first

    — b.  prone, head first

    — c.  supine, feet first

    — d.  prone, feet first

96. Which of the following cranial nerves are located in the fore-brain?

    1.    olfactory

    2.    optic

    3.    oculomotor

    — a.  1 and 2

    — b.  1 and 3

    — c.  2 and 3

    — d.  1, 2, & 3

97. Which of the following procedures would require the use of a computed tomography stereotactic guidance system?

    1.    biopsy of a brain tumor

    2.    pre-surgical localization of a brain tumor

    3.    radiation therapy planning of a brain tumor

    — a.  1 and 2

    — b.  1 and 3

    — c.  2 and 3

    — d.  1, 2, & 3

98. What filter selection would provide the best detail for imaging of the internal auditory canals?

    — a.  smooth

    — b.  standard

    — c.  sharp

    — d.  soft

99. Which of the following conditions would be demonstrated by coronal images of the orbits?

1. superior orbital rim fractures
2. blow-out fractures
3. metallic foreign bodies in the orbit

___ a. 1 and 2

___ b. 1 and 3

___ c. 2 and 3

___ d. 1, 2, & 3

100. Which of the following are indications for the use of intravenous contrast media for CT imaging of a brain infarct that is two weeks old?

1. the infarct can become hyperdense with the brain
2. the infarct can become isodense with the brain
3. the infarct can become hypodense with the brain

___ a. 1 only

___ b. 2 only

___ c. 3 only

___ d. 1, 2, & 3

101. What radiographic baseline is placed twenty degrees to the scan plane when obtaining axial scans of the pediatric brain?

___ a. glabellomeatal line

___ b. canthomeatal line

___ c. orbitomeatal line

___ d. infraorbitomeatal line

102. Which of the following anatomical structures are components of the basal ganglia?

1. lentiform nucleus
2. caudate nucleus
3. claustrum

___ a. 1 and 2

___ b. 1 and 3

___ c. 2 and 3

___ d. 1, 2, & 3

103. What anatomical structure forms a roof over the posterior cranial fossa and is shaped like a tent?

    __ a. tentorium cerebelli

    __ b. falx cerebri

    __ c. pontine cistern

    __ d. pia mater

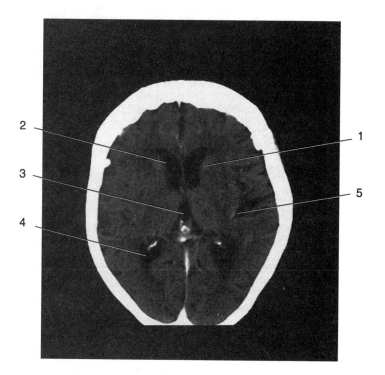

*Figure 1*

104. Which number in Figure 1 illustrates the third ventricle?

    __ a. 2

    __ b. 3

    __ c. 4

    __ d. 5

105. Which of the following is illustrated by #1 in Figure 1 ?

    __ a.  the anterior horn of the lateral ventricle

    __ b.  quadrigeminal cistern

    __ c.  thalamus

    __ d.  caudate nucleus

106. Which of the following is illustrated by #2 in Figure 1 ?

    __ a.  the anterior horn of the lateral ventricle

    __ b.  third ventricle

    __ c.  fourth ventricle

    __ d.  sylvian fissure

107. Which of the following scanning parameters should be selected for CT imaging of trauma to the maxillofacial region?

    1.  1 to 3 mm section thickness

    2.  high resolution algorithm (bone algorithm)

    3.  40cm scan field of view

    __ a.  1 and 2

    __ b.  1 and 3

    __ c.  2 and 3

    __ d.  1, 2, & 3

108. Which of the following combination of scanning parameters is preferred for assessing abnormalities within the petrous pyramids of the temporal bones?

    __ a.  wide window width, bone algorithm, 1mm to 3mm section thickness

    __ b.  narrow window width, soft tissue algorithm, 5mm to 10mm section thickness

    __ c.  wide window width, standard algorithm, 5mm to 10mm section thickness

    __ d.  narrow window width, standard algorithm 5mm to 10mm section thickness

109. Which of the following will minimize artifacts caused by dental fillings?
    1. place radiolucent sponges against the patient's head
    2. change the angle of the gantry
    3. reposition the patient's head

    ___ a. 1 and 2

    ___ b. 1 and 3

    ___ c. 2 and 3

    ___ d. 1, 2, & 3

110. What scanning plane is most effective in demonstrating the anatomical relationship between the pituitary gland and the sella turcica?

    ___ a. axial

    ___ b. coronal

    ___ c. sagittal

    ___ d. off axis oblique

111. Which of the following results from a fracture in the temporal region of the skull with associated tearing of the middle meningeal artery?

    ___ a. subdural hematoma

    ___ b. epidural hematoma

    ___ c. arteriovenous malformation

    ___ d. subarachnoid hematoma

112. Which of the following best describes the Circle of Willis?

    ___ a. separates the right and left hemispheres of the brain

    ___ b. separates the posterior fossa from the rest of the brain

    ___ c. allows communication between anterior and posterior cerebral circulation

    ___ d. connects cerebral arterial circulation with cerebral venous circulation

113. Which of the following can cause inaccurate 3D reconstructed images of the head?

    1. beam hardening artifacts
    2. metallic dental fillings
    3. patient motion

    ___ a. 1 and 2
    ___ b. 1 and 3
    ___ c. 2 and 3
    ___ d. 1, 2, & 3

114. Which of the following are directly proportional to the intensity of contrast enhancement in intracranial tumors?

    1. the amount of contrast material injected
    2. the timing of the CT images
    3. the degree of blood brain barrier breakdown

    ___ a. 1 and 2
    ___ b. 1 and 3
    ___ c. 2 and 3
    ___ d. 1, 2, & 3

115. Which of the following has the highest CT number?

    ___ a. cerebrospinal fluid
    ___ b. brain gray matter
    ___ c. brain white matter
    ___ d. calcified pituitary gland

116. What type of artifact generally appears as a dark horizontal line through the petrous ridges?

    ___ a. ring artifact
    ___ b. motion artifact
    ___ c. beam hardening artifact
    ___ d. metallic artifact

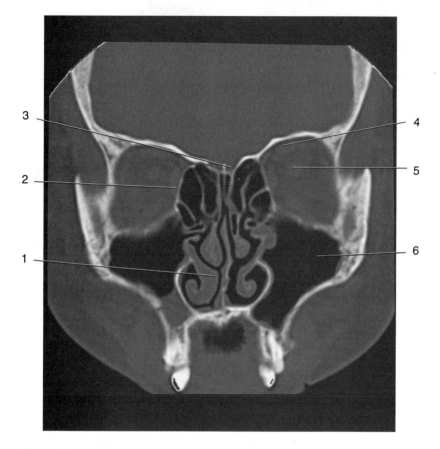

*Figure 2*

117. Which number in Figure 2 illustrates the optic nerve?

    ___ a. 2
    ___ b. 3
    ___ c. 5
    ___ d. 6

118. Which of the following is illustrated by #6 in Figure 2 ?

    ___ a. frontal sinus
    ___ b. ethmoid sinus
    ___ c. maxillary sinus
    ___ d. sphenoid sinus

119. Which of the following is illustrated by #4 in Figure 2 ?

    ___ a. optic nerve

    ___ b. inferior rectus muscle

    ___ c. lateral rectus muscle

    ___ d. superior rectus muscle

120. What canal allows communication between the third and fourth ventricles of the brain?

    ___ a. choroid plexus

    ___ b. aqueduct of Sylvius

    ___ c. foreman of Magnum

    ___ d. corpus callosum

121. Which of the following imaging sections are routinely obtained for CT scanning of the head?

1. axial
2. coronal
3. sagittal

    ___ a. 1 and 2

    ___ b. 1 and 3

    ___ c. 2 and 3

    ___ d. 1, 2, & 3

122. Which of the following are locations of cerebrospinal fluid?

1. subdural space
2. subarachnoid space
3. fourth ventricle of the brain

    ___ a. 1 and 2

    ___ b. 1 and 3

    ___ c. 2 and 3

    ___ d. 1, 2, & 3

123. Which of the following are reasons thinner section thickness is preferred for CT scanning of the posterior fossa?

    1.   reduces beam hardening artifacts
    2.   improves spatial resolution
    3.   decreases radiation dose

    __ a.   1 and 2
    __ b.   1 and 3
    __ c.   2 and 3
    __ d.   1, 2, & 3

124. Which of the following are indications for CT scanning of the head?

    1.   trauma
    2.   endocrine disease
    3.   inflammatory disease

    __ a.   1 and 2
    __ b.   1 and 3
    __ c.   2 and 3
    __ d.   1, 2, & 3

125. Which of the following cerebral abnormalities most frequently is a result of a ruptured aneurysm?

    __ a.   subarachnoid hemorrhage
    __ b.   meningioma
    __ c.   cerebral abscess
    __ d.   cerebral metastases

126. What positioning baseline is placed perpendicular to the table-top for a lateral scoutview of the head?

    __ a.   infraorbitalmeatal line
    __ b.   orbitomeatal line
    __ c.   mentomeatal line
    __ d.   acanthiomeatal line

127. Which of the following are options that can be exercised when the neck cannot be fully extended for coronal scanning of the head?

1. increase the gantry angle
2. reformation of contiguous axial scans
3. increase the scanning field of view

    ___ a. 1 and 2

    ___ b. 1 and 3

    ___ c. 2 and 3

    ___ d. 1, 2, & 3

128. Which of the following are advantages of reformatting axial images when there is trauma to the maxillofacial region?

1. it eliminates additional radiation dose to the patient
2. there is the ability to obtain off axis oblique images
3. there is the ability to obtain three dimensional images

    ___ a. 1 and 2

    ___ b. 1 and 3

    ___ c. 2 and 3

    ___ d. 1, 2, & 3

129. Which of the following anatomical regions should be included on a lateral scoutview of the paranasal sinuses?

1. base of the skull
2. midbrain region
3. top of the skull

    ___ a. 1 and 2

    ___ b. 1 and 3

    ___ c. 2 and 3

    ___ d. 1, 2, & 3

130. Which of the following scanning parameters can be increased to improve contrast resolution for CT scanning of the brain?

    1.   mA
    2.   kVp
    3.   time

    ___ a.  1 only
    ___ b.  2 only
    ___ c.  3 only
    ___ d.  1, 2, & 3

131. Where should scanning commence for routine axial CT scanning of the posterior fossa and the brain?

    ___ a.  at the level of the EAM
    ___ b.  1 cm below the EAM
    ___ c.  1 cm below the base of the skull
    ___ d.  1 cm above the base of the skull

132. Which of the following statements are true regarding axial CT of the internal auditory canals?

    1.   a scoutview is taken to include the base of the skull to the level of the third ventricle
    2.   bilateral high resolution images are obtained
    3.   the examination is performed utilizing a 1mm to 2mm section thickness

    ___ a.  1 and 2
    ___ b.  1 and 3
    ___ c.  2 and 3
    ___ d.  1, 2, & 3

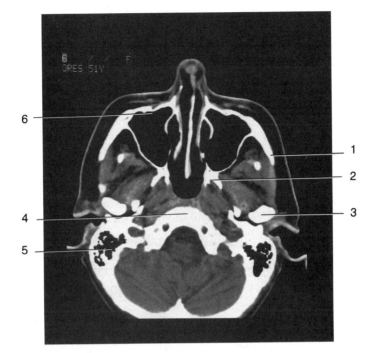

*Figure 3*

133. Which number in Figure 3 illustrates the zygomatic arch?

    ___ a. 1
    ___ b. 2
    ___ c. 3
    ___ d. 4

134. Which number in Figure 3 illustrates the mandibular condyle?

    ___ a. 2
    ___ b. 3
    ___ c. 4
    ___ d. 5

135. Which of the following is illustrated by #5 in Figure 3 ?

　　　__ a.　external auditory meatus

　　　__ b.　sphenoid sinus

　　　__ c.　mastoid air cells

　　　__ d.　zygomatic arches

## Neck                                               (#136-144)

136. What is the primary reason for having a patient phonate the letter "E" during CT examination of the larynx?

　　　__ a.　closes the pyriform sinuses

　　　__ b.　distends the laryngeal ventricles

　　　__ c.　provides definition of vocal cord mobility

　　　__ d.　provides definition of the epiglottis

137. Which of the following can be utilized to avoid dental fillings when performing a routine CT examination of the neck?

1.　gantry angulation

2.　extend the chin

3.　obtain right and left slight axial oblique projections

　　　__ a.　1 and 2

　　　__ b.　1 and 3

　　　__ c.　2 and 3

　　　__ d.　1, 2, & 3

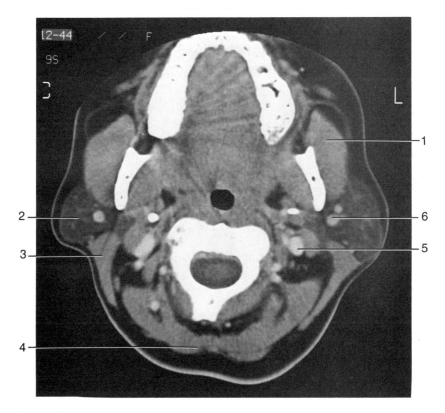

*Figure 4*

138. Which of the following is illustrated by #1 in Figure 4?

    ___ a. sternocleidomastoid muscle

    ___ b. masseter muscle

    ___ c. pterygoid muscle

    ___ d. trapezius muscle

139. Which of the following is illustrated by #6 in Figure 4?

    ___ a. internal jugular vein

    ___ b. external jugular vein

    ___ c. internal carotid artery

    ___ d. external carotid artery

140. Which of the following is illustrated by #2 in Figure 4?

___ a. submandibular gland

___ b. thyroid gland

___ c. sublingual gland

___ d. parotid gland

141. Which of the following is best assessed with axial sections that are parallel to the plane of the cervical spine and vocal cords?

___ a. nasopharynx

___ b. larynx

___ c. hard palate

___ d. masseter muscle

142. What type of scoutview is recommended for a routine CT examination of the neck?

___ a. AP

___ b. lateral

___ c. PA

___ d. oblique

143. Where does the scout view commence and conclude for a routine CT of the neck?

___ a. from T2 to the mid-brain region

___ b. from C5 to the mid-brain region

___ c. from T4 to the top of the skull

___ d. from the mandibular rami to the EAM

144. At what level does the common carotid artery bifurcate into the internal and external carotid arteries?

___ a. C1-C2

___ b. C2-C3

___ c. C4-C5

___ d. T1-T2

# Spine                                      *(#145-177)*

145. What is the region that should be covered for examination of one intervertebral disc space?

___ a. from the pedicle of the vertebra above to the pedicle of the vertebra below

___ b. from the superior articular process of the vertebra above to the inferior articular process of the vertebra below

___ c. from the spinous process of the vertebra above to the spinous process of the vertebra below

___ d. from the apophyseal joint of the vertebra above to the apophyseal joint of the vertebra below

146. How long after an injection of contrast media should a post myelogram CT scan be performed?

___ a. 2 to 6 hrs

___ b. 8 to 10 hrs

___ c. 12 hrs

___ d. 24 hrs

147. Which of the following are reasons for performing a CT of the lumbar spine with and without intravenous contrast media?

1. to visualize the dura and blood vessels
2. to visualize a herniated disc
3. to differentiate surgical scar tissue adjacent to the spinal cord spinal cord

___ a. 1 and 2

___ b. 1 and 3

___ c. 2 and 3

___ d. 1, 2, & 3

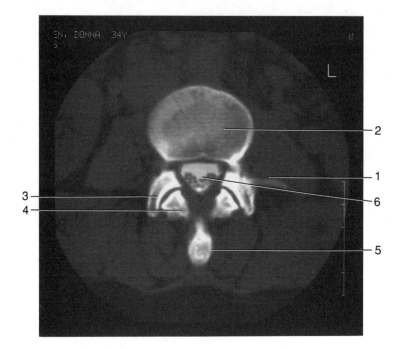

*Figure 5*

148. Which of the following is illustrated by #3 in Figure 5?

___ a. transverse process

___ b. superior articular process

___ c. inferior articular process

___ d. spinous process

149. Which of the following is illustrated by #1 in Figure 5?

___ a. transverse process

___ b. superior articular process

___ c. inferior articular process

___ d. spinous process

150. Which of the following is illustrated by #5 in Figure 5?

___ a. transverse process

___ b. spinous process

___ c. ligamentum flavum

___ d. dural sac

151. How are axial sections angled for most spine exams?

___ a.   parallel to the spinous process

___ b.   parallel to the body

___ c.   parallel to each disk space

___ d.   parallel to the apophyseal joints

152. At what vertebral level does the spinal cord terminate in the adult?

___ a.   T12-L1

___ b.   L2-L3

___ c.   L4-L5

___ d.   at the second sacral segment

153. Where is contrast media introduced for a myelography examination of the spinal canal?

___ a.   the subdural space

___ b.   the epidural space

___ c.   the subarachnoid space

___ d.   the spinal cord

154. Which of the following combinations of section thickness and table incrementation are recommended for CT scanning of the cervical spine when assessing disk disease?

___ a.   2mm section thickness, 5mm incrementation

___ b.   5mm section thickness, 5mm incrementation

___ c.   3mm section thickness, 2mm incrementation

___ d.   5mm section thickness, 10mm incrementation

155. Which of the following are advantages of CT of the spine verses myelography?

   1. CT is more sensitive and precise for the assessment of lateral disk herniation

   2. CT can diagnose intrathecal abnormalities better than myelography (intradural tumors)

   3. CT is more useful for lesions of the cervicothoracic region

     \_\_ a. 1 only

     \_\_ b. 2 only

     \_\_ c. 3 only

     \_\_ d. 1, 2, & 3

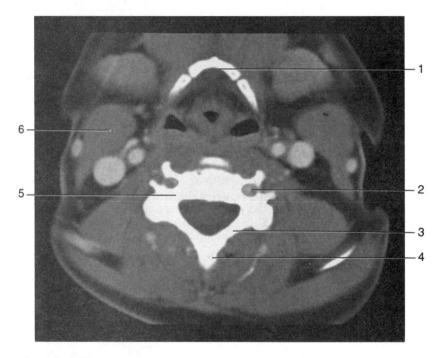

*Figure 6*

156. What anatomical structure is illustrated by #1 in Figure 6?

     \_\_ a. thyroid cartilage

     \_\_ b. cricoid cartilage

     \_\_ c. hyoid bone

     \_\_ d. mandible

157. What number in Figure 6 illustrates the lamina of the cervical vertebrae?

___ a. 2

___ b. 3

___ c. 4

___ d. 5

158. Which of the following is illustrated by #5 in Figure 6?

___ a. the lamina of a cervical vertebrae

___ b. the pedicle of a cervical vertebrae

___ c. the spinous process of a cervical vertebrae

___ d. the body of a cervical vertebrae

159. Which of the following is illustrated by #2 in Figure 6?

___ a. intervertebral foreman

___ b. transverse foreman

___ c. spinal cord

___ d. internal carotid artery

160. What should the technologist do in positioning of the supine patient to decrease the lordotic curvature of the lumbar spine?

___ a. extend the legs equally

___ b. flex the knees over a small foam wedge

___ c. flex the knees and have the patient hold their knees

___ d. flex the knees over a large foam wedge

161. Which of the following are indications for computed tomography of the spine?

1. suspected spinal stenosis
2. suspected spinal infection
3. suspected intraspinal tumor

___ a. 1 and 2

___ b. 1 and 3

___ c. 2 and 3

___ d. 1, 2, & 3

162. What are the best breathing instructions for the patient during an exam of the spine?

___ a.  deep inspiration with suspension during the scan

___ b.  full exhalation with suspension during the scan

___ c.  suspend respiration during scan

___ d.  equal inspiration with suspension during the scan

163. Which of the following CT findings are possible indicators of a herniated disc?

1.  displacement of epidural fat
2.  hypertrophy of the inferior articulating process and lamina
3.  deformity of the posterior border of the disc

___ a.  1 and 2

___ b.  1 and 3

___ c.  2 and 3

___ d.  1, 2, & 3

164. Which of the following scanning planes when reformatted from the axial plane would best demonstrate the degree of extension of a vertebral mass into the spinal canal?

1.  coronal
2.  sagittal
3.  oblique

___ a.  1 only

___ b.  2 only

___ c.  3 only

___ d.  1, 2, & 3

165. Which type of scout view is used for cervical spine exams?

___ a.  AP

___ b.  PA

___ c.  lateral

___ d.  oblique

166. Which of the following are reasons for the operator to select a displayed field of view that is smaller than the scanned field of view for imaging of the spine in the axial plane?

    1. spatial resolution is increased
    2. the operators perceptibility of detail is increased
    3. the actual displayed image detail is increased

    ___ a.  1 and 2
    ___ b.  1 and 3
    ___ c.  2 and 3
    ___ d.  1, 2, & 3

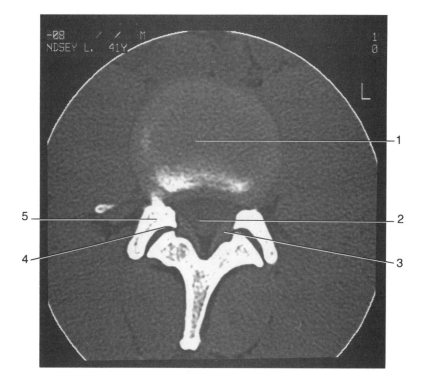

*Figure 7*

167. Which of the following is illustrated by #3 in Figure 7?

    ___ a.  intertransverse ligament
    ___ b.  ligamentum flavum
    ___ c.  ligamentum teres
    ___ d.  ligamentum nuchae

168. Which of the following is illustrated by #4 in Figure 7?

___ a.  costovertebral joint

___ b.  apophyseal joint

___ c.  intervertebral joint

___ d.  costotransverse joint

169. Which of the following is illustrated by #1 in Figure 7?

___ a.  vertebral body

___ b.  intervertebral disk

___ c.  spinal cord

___ d.  intervertebral foreman

170. What can be done to prevent artifacts from contrast media layering in the intrathecal space?

___ a.  roll the patient two or three times before scanning

___ b.  place the patient's head lower than the body

___ c.  raise the patient's head higher than the body

___ d.  drain the contrast media from the patient

171. Which of the following scanning acquisition methods can be utilized for CT scanning of the spine?

1.  high resolution computed tomography
2.  helical/spiral computed tomography
3.  dynamic computed tomography

___ a.  1 only

___ b.  2 only

___ c.  3 only

___ d.  1, 2, & 3

172. Which of the following scanning acquisition methods would allow reconstruction through the middle of a intraspinal tumor at 0.1mm increments?

 1. high resolution computed tomography
 2. helical/spiral computed tomography
 3. dynamic computed tomography

   __ a. 1 only

   __ b. 2 only

   __ c. 3 only

   __ d. 1, 2, & 3

173. Which of the following may help to show areas of disc herniation in the cervical spine?

 1. intravenous contrast
 2. negative (air) contrast
 3. intrathecal contrast

   __ a. 1 and 2

   __ b. 1 and 3

   __ c. 2 and 3

   __ d. 1, 2, & 3

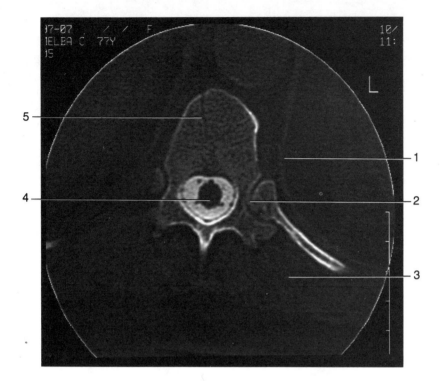

*Figure 8*

174. Which of the following is illustrated by #3 in Figure 8?

___ a. psoas muscle

___ b. trapezius muscle

___ c. posterior oblique muscle

___ d. erector spinae muscle

175. Which of the following is illustrated by #2 in Figure 8?

___ a. costovertebral joint

___ b. costotransverse joint

___ c. apophyseal joint

___ d. intervertebral joint

176. Which of the following is illustrated by #5 in Figure 8?

    \_\_ a.  longitudinal fracture

    \_\_ b.  spinal nerve

    \_\_ c.  vascular groove

    \_\_ d.  intervertebral joint space

177. Which of the following is illustrated by #1 in Figure 8?

    \_\_ a.  psoas muscle

    \_\_ b.  spinal artery

    \_\_ c.  spinal nerve

    \_\_ d.  crus of the diaphragm

# Chest                                                        *(#178-222)*

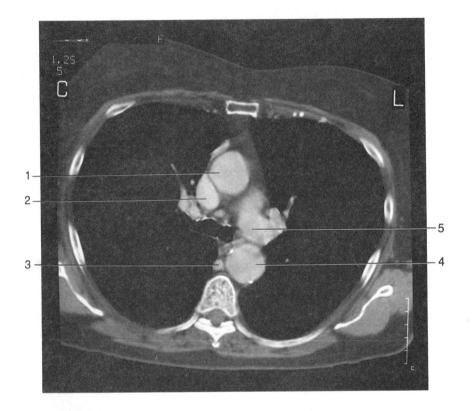

*Figure 9*

178. Which of the following is illustrated by #2 in Figure 9?

    ___ a.  ascending aorta

    ___ b.  descending aorta

    ___ c.  superior vena cava

    ___ d.  inferior vena cava

179. Which of the following is illustrated by #3 in Figure 9?

    \_\_ a.  azygos vein

    \_\_ b.  pulmonary artery

    \_\_ c.  esophagus

    \_\_ d.  lymph node

180. Which of the following is illustrated by #4 in Figure 9?

    \_\_ a.  ascending aorta

    \_\_ b.  descending aorta

    \_\_ c.  inferior vena cava

    \_\_ d.  esophagus

181. Which of the following is the typical method for filming of routine chest exams?

    1.  windowed to show mediastinal structures
    2.  windowed to show lung structures
    3.  windowed to show bony structures

    \_\_ a.  1 and 2

    \_\_ b.  1 and 3

    \_\_ c.  2 and 3

    \_\_ d.  1, 2, & 3

182. Which of the following are advantages of contrast enhancement of thorax?

    1.  allows the differentiation of aortic aneurysms from mediastinal masses
    2.  defines the presence and extent of traumatic aneurysms
    3.  aids in the determination of the relationship of a mass to surrounding structures and extension into the mediastinum

    \_\_ a.  1 and 2

    \_\_ b.  1 and 3

    \_\_ c.  2 and 3

    \_\_ d.  1, 2, & 3

183. What is the scan extent for CT of the chest when lung carcinoma is suspected?

    ___ a. from the root of the neck through the adrenal glands

    ___ b. from the sternal notch to the lower poles of the kidney

    ___ c. from the clavicles to the mid liver region

    ___ d. from the sternal notch to the base of the heart

184. Which of the following is the suggested amount and delivery rate of contrast media that is necessary to optimally visualize the vasculature of the mediastinum when the bolus method is solely used?

    ___ a. 5 seconds per 50ml of contrast media

    ___ b. 5 seconds per 100ml of contrast media

    ___ c. 10 seconds per 50ml of contrast media

    ___ d. 10 seconds per 200ml of contrast media

185. Which of the following scout views are recommended for routine chest exams?

    ___ a. a frontal projection from the clavicles to the base of the heart

    ___ b. a lateral projection from the root of the neck to the upper abdomen

    ___ c. a frontal projection from the root of the neck to the upper abdomen

    ___ d. a lateral projection from the clavicles to the base of the heart

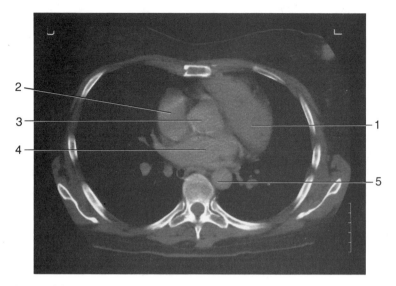

*Figure 10*

186. What anatomical structure is illustrated by #4 in Figure 10?

___ a. left ventricle of the heart

___ b. right ventricle of the heart

___ c. left atrium of the heart

___ d. right atrium of the heart

187. Which of the following is illustrated by #3 in Figure 10?

___ a. superior vena cava

___ b. ascending aorta

___ c. descending aorta

___ d. pulmonary artery

188. Which of the following is illustrated by #1 in Figure 10?

___ a. left ventricle of the heart

___ b. pulmonary trunk

___ c. ascending aorta

___ d. left atrium of the heart

189. What is the most substantial risk involved in an aspiration biopsy of a chest lesion?

___ a.  pneumonia

___ b.  hematoma

___ c.  pneumothorax

___ d.  allergic reaction

190. Which of the following are considered to be part of the mediastinum?

1.  heart
2.  the great vessels
3.  thymus

___ a.  1 and 2

___ b.  1 and 3

___ c.  2 and 3

___ d.  1, 2, & 3

191. What is the usual position of the patient for studies of the chest?

___ a.  supine

___ b.  prone

___ c.  right lateral decubitus

___ d.  left lateral decubitus

192. Which of the following statements regarding the pleural cavity are true?

1.  air moves freely in and out during respiration
2.  the right and left pleural cavities are separate and closed
3.  it is a potential space between the layers of the pleura

___ a.  1 and 2

___ b.  1 and 3

___ c.  2 and 3

___ d.  1, 2, & 3

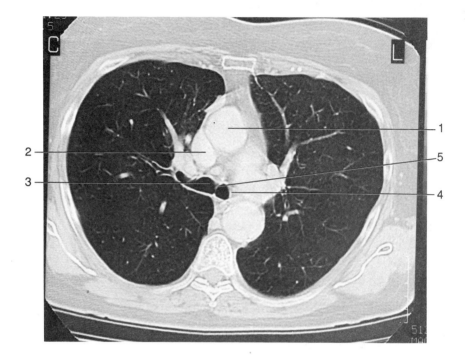

*Figure 11*

193. Which number in Figure 11 represents the right mainstem bronchus?

    ___ a.  1
    ___ b.  2
    ___ c.  3
    ___ d.  5

194. Which of the following is illustrated by #5 in Figure 11?

    ___ a.  azygos vein
    ___ b.  carina
    ___ c.  secondary bronchial division
    ___ d.  pericardial septum

195. Which of the following illustrated by #2 in Figure 11?

  ___ a. superior vena cava

  ___ b. inferior vena cava

  ___ c. azygos vein

  ___ d. ascending aorta

196. Which of the following could be used to avoid reaching the x-ray tube heat capacity limit when performing dynamic scanning of the thorax?

  1. lower mAs
  2. select half scan mode before beginning
  3. only use the dynamic sequence through the mediastinum and hila.

  ___ a. 1 and 2

  ___ b. 1 and 3

  ___ c. 2 and 3

  ___ d. 1, 2, & 3

197. Which of the following CT acquisition methods can produce high resolution images of the heart?

  1. conventional
  2. dynamic scanning
  3. ultrafast CT (electron beam)

  ___ a. 1 only

  ___ b. 2 only

  ___ c. 3 only

  ___ d. 1, 2, & 3

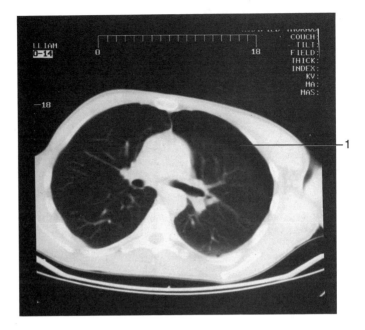

*Figure 12*

198. What type of pathology is illustrated by #1 in Figure 12?

___ a. atelectasis

___ b. pneumonia

___ c. pneumothorax

___ d. lung carcinoma

199. Which of the following window widths and window levels would best correlate with Figure 12?

___ a. 1600/WW, 600/WL

___ b. -160/WW, 600/WL

___ c. -1600/WW, -600/WL

___ d. 1600/WW, -600/WL

200. Which of the following are causes of pleural effusion?

    1.    increased capillary pressure as in congestive heart failure

    2.    increased negative intrapleural pressure which develops with atelectasis

    3.    impaired lymphatic drainage of the pleural space

    ___ a.  1 and 2

    ___ b.  1 and 3

    ___ c.  2 and 3

    ___ d.  1, 2, & 3

201. What type of artifact is caused by selecting a scanned field of view that is smaller than the patients thorax measurement?

    ___ a.  edge gradient artifact

    ___ b.  out of field artifact

    ___ c.  ring artifact

    ___ d.  motion artifact

202. Where are the arms placed during exams of the chest?

    ___ a.  to the patient's sides

    ___ b.  on the patient's chest

    ___ c.  above the patient's head

    ___ d.  under the patients head

203. Which of the following medical laboratory tests should be performed prior to performing a CT guided biopsy of the lung?

    1.    prothrombin time

    2.    partial prothrombin time

    3.    platelet count

    ___ a.  1 and 2

    ___ b.  1 and 3

    ___ c.  2 and 3

    ___ d.  1, 2, & 3

204. Which of the following statements regarding the superior vena cava are true?

 1. SVC receives blood from the azygos vein
 2. SVC drains into the right atrium
 3. SVC is formed by the union of the right and left pulmonary veins

        ___ a. 1 and 2

        ___ b. 1 and 3

        ___ c. 2 and 3

        ___ d. 1, 2, & 3

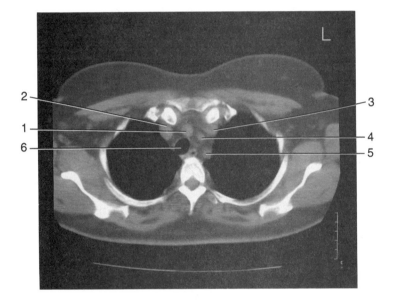

*Figure 13*

205. What number in Figure 13 illustrates the right brachiocephalic vein?

        ___ a. 1

        ___ b. 2

        ___ c. 5

        ___ d. 6

206. Which of the following is illustrated by #6 in Figure 13?

  ___ a. esophagus

  ___ b. right mainstem bronchus

  ___ c. trachea

  ___ d. thyroid

207. Which of the following is illustrated by #4 in Figure 13?

  ___ a. lymph node

  ___ b. brachiocephalic artery

  ___ c. common carotid artery

  ___ d. brachiocephalic vein

208. Which of the following window widths and window levels would best demonstrate mediastinal anatomy?

  ___ a. 1400 WW, -400 WL

  ___ b. -1400 WW, 400 WL

  ___ c. 400 WW, 50 WL

  ___ d. -400 WW, -50 WL

209. Which of the following is characterized by an intimal flap displaced inward dividing the aorta into true and false channels?

  ___ a. saccular aneurysm

  ___ b. fusiform aneurysm

  ___ c. berry aneurysm

  ___ d. dissecting aneurysm

210. Which of the following are indications for computed tomography of the thorax?

  1. detection of pulmonary masses
  2. to determine if a pulmonary infiltrate is an abscess
  3. to define pleural tumor extent

  ___ a. 1 and 2

  ___ b. 1 and 3

  ___ c. 2 and 3

  ___ d. 1, 2, & 3

211. What is a typical section thickness for routine survey studies of the chest?

    __ a.  1-2 mm

    __ b.  3-5 mm

    __ c.  5-8 mm

    __ d.  8-10 mm

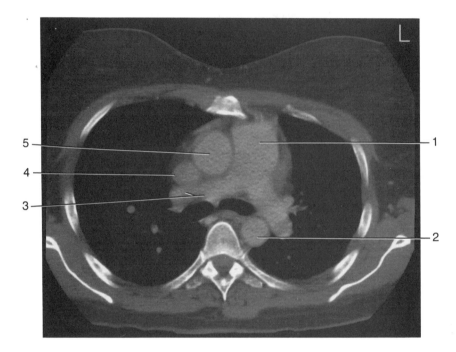

*Figure 14*

212. Which of the following is illustrated by #3 in Figure 14?

    __ a.  superior vena cava

    __ b.  inferior vena cava

    __ c.  descending aorta

    __ d.  pulmonary artery

213. Which of the following is illustrated by #1 in Figure 14?

 __ a. left ventricle of the heart

 __ b. ascending aorta

 __ c. descending aorta

 __ d. pulmonary trunk

214. Which of the following is illustrated by #4 in Figure 14?

 __ a. ascending aorta

 __ b. descending aorta

 __ c. superior vena cava

 __ d. inferior vena cava

215. Which of the following breathing instructions should be used for routine scanning of the chest?

 __ a. deep inspiration and hold

 __ b. exhalation and hold

 __ c. suspend respiration as scan begins

 __ d. standard inspiration and hold

216. Which of the following are components of the high resolution computed tomography technique used for imaging of the lung parenchyma?

 1. high spatial frequency algorithm that enhances edge detection
 2. 10mm section thickness
 3. decreased displayed field of view

 __ a. 1 and 2

 __ b. 1 and 3

 __ c. 2 and 3

 __ d. 1, 2, & 3

217. Which of the following is the recommended injection site to introduce contrast media for CT examination of the chest?

 __ a. right arm in a laterally situated antecubital vein

 __ b. right arm in a medially situated antecubital vein

 __ c. left arm in a laterally situated antecubital vein

 __ d. left arm in a medially situated antecubital vein

218. Which of the following are advantages of helical/spiral scanning compared to dynamic sequential scanning of the thorax?

   1. elimination of an interscan and intergroup delay

   2. artifacts due to patient motion are reduced

   3. greater accuracy in multiplanar reconstruction and 3D processing is possible

   ___ a. 1 and 2

   ___ b. 1 and 3

   ___ c. 2 and 3

   ___ d. 1, 2, & 3

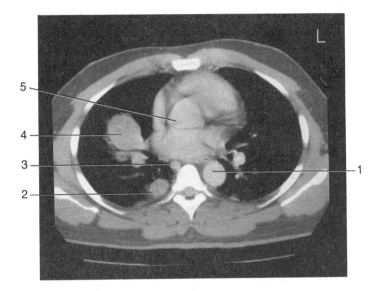

*Figure 15*

219. Which of the following is illustrated by #2 in Figure 15?

   ___ a. psoas muscle

   ___ b. descending aorta

   ___ c. pathological process

   ___ d. lymph node

220. Which of the following is illustrated by #4 in Figure 15?

    __ a.  superior vena cava

    __ b.  pathological process

    __ c.  ascending aorta

    __ d.  descending aorta

221. Which of the following is illustrated by #1 in Figure 15?

    __ a.  ascending aorta

    __ b.  descending aorta

    __ c.  thorax pathology

    __ d.  lymph node

222. Which of the following are superficial muscles of the thorax?

1.    pectoralis major

2.    trapezius

3.    latissimus dorsi

    __ a.  1 and 2

    __ b.  1 and 3

    __ c.  2 and 3

    __ d.  1, 2, & 3

# Abdomen                   (#223-267)

223. Which of the following oral contrast administrations would be used for a routine abdomen exam?

1.    300-500 ml given 1 to 2 hours prior to the exam

2.    300-500 ml given immediately prior to the exam

3.    300-500 ml given at least 4-6 hours prior to the exam

    __ a.  1 and 2

    __ b.  1 and 3

    __ c.  2 and 3

    __ d.  1, 2, & 3

224. Which of the following is the recommended percentage of barium in a barium sulfate suspension utilized in abdominal computed tomography?

___ a. 1-3%

___ b. 6-10%

___ c. 15-20%

___ d. 40%

225. What is the recommended percentage of a water soluble contrast agent in a prepared mixture for abdominal computed tomography?

___ a. 1-3%

___ b. 6-10%

___ c. 15-20%

___ d. 40%

226. Which of the following statements are true regarding the administration of oral contrast media for abdominal computed tomography?

1. provides adequate luminal distention necessary to estimate wall thickness
2. aids in distinguishing a loop of bowel from an abnormal fluid collection
3. aids in distinguishing a loop of bowel from an abdominal mass

___ a. 1 and 2

___ b. 1 and 3

___ c. 2 and 3

___ d. 1, 2, & 3

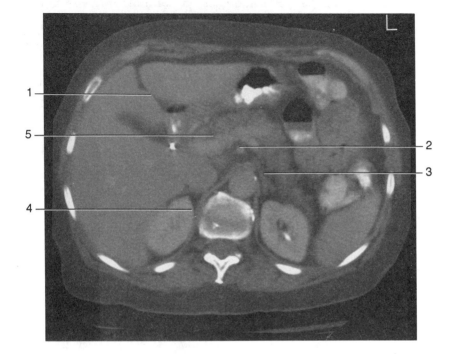

*Figure 16*

227. Which of the following is illustrated by # 1 in Figure 16?

___ a. ligamentum teres

___ b. portal vein

___ c. hepatic artery

___ d. common bile duct

228. Which of the following is illustrated by # 3 in Figure 16?

___ a. renal artery

___ b. adrenal gland

___ c. splenic artery

___ d. crus of the diaphragm

229. Which of the following is illustrated by # 2 in Figure 16?

    ___ a. inferior mesenteric artery

    ___ b. superior mesenteric artery

    ___ c. suprarenal artery

    ___ d. gastric artery

230. Which of the following areas should be covered for a scout view of the abdomen?

    ___ a. from the angle of the ribs to the bottom of the kidneys

    ___ b. from the superior bases of the lungs to the iliac crest

    ___ c. from the heart to the symphysis pubis

    ___ d. from the top of the kidneys to the bottom of the bladder

231. Which of the following are retroperitoneal structures?

1. pancreas
2. duodenum
3. kidneys

    ___ a. 1 and 2

    ___ b. 1 and 3

    ___ c. 2 and 3

    ___ d. 1, 2, & 3

232. Which of the following are indications for abdominal percutaneous needle biopsy?

1. localizing an intraabdominal lesion
2. determining the nature of an abnormality
3. staging of intraabdominal malignancies

    ___ a. 1 and 2

    ___ b. 1 and 3

    ___ c. 2 and 3

    ___ d. 1, 2, & 3

233. In which of the following time frames does maximum opacification of the medullary portion of the kidneys occur after an injection of intravenous contrast media?

   ___ a. 10 to 30 seconds

   ___ b. 1 to 3 minutes

   ___ c. 5 to 8 minutes

   ___ d. 10 minutes

234. What is an acceptable initial dose of intravenous contrast media for CT evaluation of the pediatric abdomen?

   ___ a. 1-2ml/kg

   ___ b. 5-10ml/kg

   ___ c. 12-15ml/kg

   ___ d. 50ml/kg

235. Which of the following can cause artifacts that make visualization of the adrenal glands difficult?

1. respiratory motion
2. bowel peristalsis
3. surgical clips

   ___ a. 1 and 2

   ___ b. 1 and 3

   ___ c. 2 and 3

   ___ d. 1, 2, & 3

236. Which of the following are phases of vascular contrast enhancement that occur following a sustained bolus injection of contrast media ?

1. bolus phase
2. nonequilibrium phase
3. equilibrium phase

   ___ a. 1 and 2

   ___ b. 1 and 3

   ___ c. 2 and 3

   ___ d. 1, 2, & 3

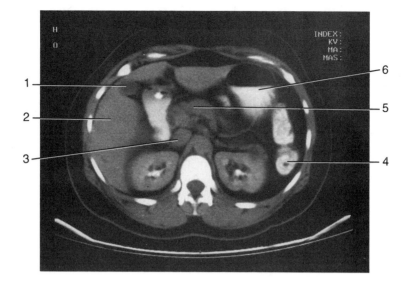

*Figure 17*

237. Which of the following is illustrated by #4 in Figure 17?

 ___ a. hepatic flexure of the colon

 ___ b. splenic flexure of the colon

 ___ c. jejunum

 ___ d. ileum

238. What number in Figure 17 illustrates the gallbladder?

 ___ a. 1

 ___ b. 2

 ___ c. 3

 ___ d. 4

239. Which of the following is illustrated by #6 in Figure 17?

 ___ a. ascending colon

 ___ b. descending colon

 ___ c. stomach

 ___ d. duodenum

240. Which of the following are techniques that can aid in the detection of liver lesions?

    1.    rescan the patient 4 to 6 hours following administration of a full dose of contrast media

    2.    refilm the case using a narrow window width

    3.    use a bolus injection technique with rapid sequential scanning

    ___ a.  1 only

    ___ b.  2 only

    ___ c.  3 only

    ___ d.  1, 2, & 3

241. What phase of respiration should be utilized for routine abdominal computed tomography?

    ___ a.  relaxed suspended inspiration

    ___ b.  relaxed suspended expiration

    ___ c.  forced expiration

    ___ d.  shallow breathing

242. Which of the following unite to form the common bile duct?

    1.    common hepatic duct

    2.    pancreatic duct

    3.    cystic duct

    ___ a.  1 and 2

    ___ b.  1 and 3

    ___ c.  2 and 3

    ___ d.  1, 2, & 3

243. Which of the following section thicknesses and couch intervals are recommended for routine CT scanning of the pancreas?

    ___ a.  5mm section thickness, 5mm couch interval

    ___ b.  5mm section thickness, 10mm couch interval

    ___ c.  10mm section thickness, 10mm couch interval

    ___ d.  10mm section thickness, 20mm couch interval

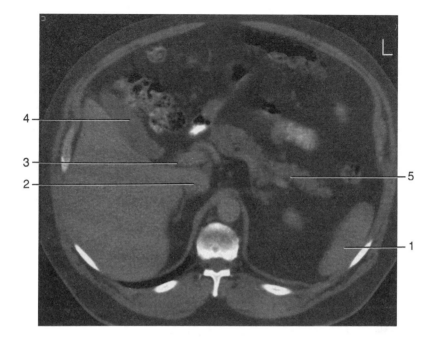

*Figure 18*

244. Which of the following is illustrated by #3 in Figure 18?

_____ a. inferior vena cava

_____ b. head of the pancreas

_____ c. portal vein

_____ d. portal artery

245. Which of the following is illustrated by #5 in Figure 18?

_____ a. head of the pancreas

_____ b. tail of the pancreas

_____ c. splenic vein

_____ d. splenic artery

246. Which of the following is illustrated by #1 in Figure 18?

    ___ a.  kidney

    ___ b.  spleen

    ___ c.  pancreas

    ___ d.  descending colon

247. In which of the following positions can the patient placed if the pancreatic boundaries are not visualized during supine scanning?

    1.  prone
    2.  left lateral decubitus
    3.  right lateral decubitus

    ___ a.  1 only

    ___ b.  2 only

    ___ c.  3 only

    ___ d.  1, 2, & 3

248. Why is computed tomography superior to ultrasound when the retroperitoneum is being evaluated?

    ___ a.  the retroperitoneum is often obscured on ultrasound due to bowel gas and fat

    ___ b.  ultrasound cannot differentiate a solid mass from a cystic mass

    ___ c.  ultrasound cannot be used for aspiration procedures

    ___ d.  the retroperitoneum is too large for ultrasound to evaluate

249. Which of the following would increase the contrast resolution of structures located in the abdomen?

    1.  decrease the mAs
    2.  selection of a low spatial frequency algorithm
    3.  decrease the section thickness

    ___ a.  1 and 2

    ___ b.  1 and 3

    ___ c.  2 and 3

    ___ d.  1, 2, & 3

250. Which of the following are benign lesions of the liver?

1. hemangioma
2. adenoma
3. adenocarcinoma

___ a. 1 and 2

___ b. 1 and 3

___ c. 2 and 3

___ d. 1, 2, & 3

251. Which of following vessels can contrast media be introduced for CT arteriography and CT arterial portography to detect liver lesions?

1. inferior vena cava
2. superior mesenteric artery
3. hepatic artery

___ a. 1 and 2

___ b. 1 and 3

___ c. 2 and 3

___ d. 1, 2, & 3

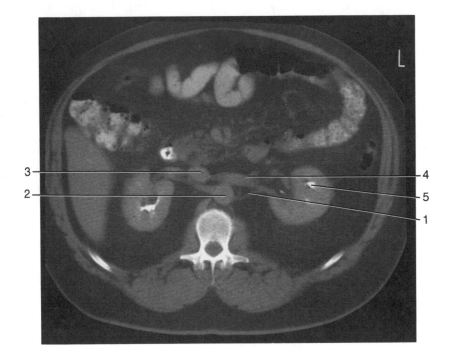

*Figure 19*

252. Which of the following is illustrated by #1 in Figure 19?

    ___ a. renal artery

    ___ b. renal vein

    ___ c. ureter

    ___ d. splenic artery

253. Which of the following is illustrated by #4 in Figure 19?

    ___ a. renal artery

    ___ b. renal vein

    ___ c. ureter

    ___ d. splenic artery

254. Which of the following is illustrated by #2 in Figure 19?

___ a. inferior mesenteric artery

___ b. superior mesenteric artery

___ c. inferior vena cava

___ d. abdominal aorta

255. Which of the following are reasons that a patient should be kept NPO after midnight the night before a CT examination of the abdomen?

1. minimize vomiting and aspiration if intravenous contrast media is used

2. to avoid diagnostic confusion between intragastric masses and ingested food

3. to make it easier for the patient to ingest the oral contrast

___ a. 1 and 2

___ b. 1 and 3

___ c. 2 and 3

___ d. 1, 2, & 3

256. What is the primary purpose for obtaining a pre-intravenous contrast abdominal scan?

___ a. pre-contrast scans are obtained to evaluate and determine specific levels prior to a dynamic scanning technique

___ b. to visualize portal circulation

___ c. to maximize lesion detection

___ d. to differentiate a loop of bowel from an intraabdominal mass

257. Which of the following CT acquisition methods would provide the best results in the shortest amount of time for trauma abdominal scanning?

___ a. high resolution computed tomography

___ b. dynamic scanning computed tomography

___ c. helical/spiral computed tomography

___ d. conventional computed tomography

258. Which of the following are methods by which malignant neoplasms metastasize?

1.   seeding within body cavities
2.   lymphatic spread
3.   embolistic spread

    ___ a.   1 and 2

    ___ b.   1 and 3

    ___ c.   2 and 3

    ___ d.   1, 2, & 3

259. Which of the following would be visualized first when coronal images are obtained via multiplanar reformation from posterior to anterior?

    ___ a.   neck of the pancreas

    ___ b.   transverse colon

    ___ c.   stomach

    ___ d.   spleen

260. Which of the following structures is most anterior?

    ___ a.   head of the pancreas

    ___ b.   inferior vena cava

    ___ c.   right adrenal gland

    ___ d.   left kidney

261. Which of the following anatomical structures would be visualized first when obtaining sagittal sections from right to left?

    ___ a.   c-loop of the duodenum

    ___ b.   tail of the pancreas

    ___ c.   gallbladder

    ___ d.   right kidney

262. Which of the following join to form the portal vein?

1. splenic vein
2. superior mesenteric vein
3. celiac vein

___ a. 1 and 2
___ b. 1 and 3
___ c. 2 and 3
___ d. 1, 2, & 3

263. Which of the following can be detected by computed tomography following blunt trauma to the abdomen?

1. fracture of the kidney
2. subcapsular hematoma of the spleen
3. retroperitoneal hemorrhage

___ a. 1 and 2
___ b. 1 and 3
___ c. 2 and 3
___ d. 1, 2, & 3

264. Which of the following are difficulties that can be encountered during CT scanning of the spleen following abdominal trauma?

1. streak artifacts can be caused by the adjacent ribs
2. lack of homogenous splenic opacification with contrast enhancement
3. streak artifacts from oral contrast media can obscure the spleen

___ a. 1 and 2
___ b. 1 and 3
___ c. 2 and 3
___ d. 1, 2, & 3

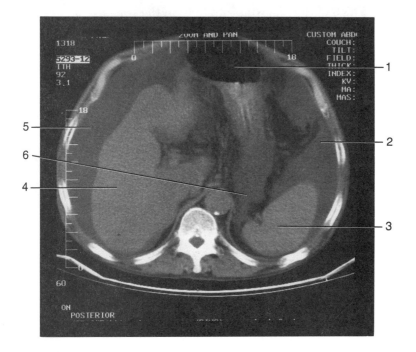

*Figure 20*

265. Which of the following is illustrated by #1 in Figure 20?

___ a. peritoneal abscess

___ b. intraabdominal hematoma

___ c. intraabdominal hemorrhage

___ d. fundus of the stomach

266. If #5 in Figure 20 has an attenuation value of 3.5, which of the following is most likely demonstrated?

___ a. ascites

___ b. hemorrhage

___ c. liver tissue

___ d. pneumoperitoneum

267. Which of the following is illustrated by #3 in Figure 20?

___ a. left kidney

___ b. spleen

___ c. hematoma

___ d. hemorrhage

# Pelvis                                                    *(#268-303)*

268. What is the scan extent for a routine survey of the pelvis?

___ a.   iliac crests to the symphysis pubis

___ b.   iliac crests to the rectum

___ c.   lung bases to the iliac crests

___ d.   lung bases to the symphysis pubis

269. What anatomical structure appears as an oval structure indenting the posterior aspect of the bladder in the female pelvis in the axial plane?

___ a.   rectum

___ b.   vagina

___ c.   uterus

___ d.   sacrum

270. Which of the following are reasons a tampon is inserted into the female vagina for CT scanning of the pelvis?

1.   identification of the vaginal canal
2.   localize the cervix and uterus
3.   replaces the use of intravenous contrast media

___ a.   1 and 2

___ b.   1 and 3

___ c.   2 and 3

___ d.   1, 2, & 3

271. Which of the following are acceptable methods of oral contrast administration for visualization of the distal colon?

1.   500 cc's of contrast administered orally the night prior to the examination
2.   300-500 cc's of contrast administered rectally just prior to the examination
3.   300-500 cc's of contrast administered orally 30 minutes prior to the examination

___ a.   1 and 2

___ b.   1 and 3

___ c.   2 and 3

___ d.   1, 2, & 3

272. Which of the following would provide the best information when suspicious densities are seen about the pelvic floor on axial scans?

   ___ a. coronal image reformation

   ___ b. sagittal image reformation

   ___ c. direct coronal scanning

   ___ d. direct decubitus scanning

273. Which of the following structures are contained within the scrotum of the male?

1. epididymis
2. seminal vesicles
3. testes

   ___ a. 1 and 2

   ___ b. 1 and 3

   ___ c. 2 and 3

   ___ d. 1, 2, & 3

274. Which of the following statements about the vasculature of the pelvis are true?

1. common iliac arteries divide into the internal and external iliac arteries
2. the internal iliac artery is the largest artery in the pelvis
3. the abdominal aorta bifurcates into the right and left common iliac arteries at the L4 vertebral level

   ___ a. 1 and 2

   ___ b. 1 and 3

   ___ c. 2 and 3

   ___ d. 1, 2, & 3

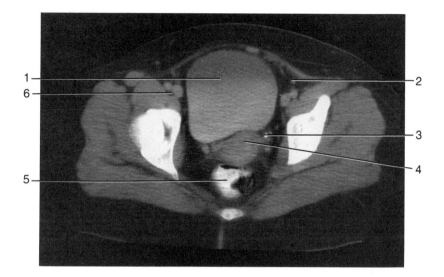

*Figure 21*

275. Which of the following is illustrated by #6 in Figure 21?

___ a.  external iliac artery

___ b.  external iliac vein

___ c.  pelvic lymph node

___ d.  ureter

276. Which of the following is illustrated by #3 in Figure 21?

___ a.  external iliac artery

___ b.  external iliac vein

___ c.  pelvic lymph node

___ d.  ureter

277. What number illustrates the urinary bladder in Figure 21?

___ a.  1

___ b.  3

___ c.  4

___ d.  5

278. Which of the following are acceptable methods of contrast media introduction for CT scanning of the urinary bladder?

    1.   iodinated contrast media given intravenously
    2.   iodinated contrast media introduced via Foley catheter
    3.   carbon dioxide introduced via Foley catheter

    ___ a.   1 and 2
    ___ b.   1 and 3
    ___ c.   2 and 3
    ___ d.   1, 2, & 3

279. In which of the following conditions would computed tomography be selected in place of ultrasound as the modality of choice when examining the pelvis?

    1.   evaluation of the extent of a known malignancy
    2.   routine diagnosis of a gynecological abnormality
    3.   pelvic abscess that contains gas

    ___ a.   1 and 2
    ___ b.   1 and 3
    ___ c.   2 and 3
    ___ d.   1, 2, & 3

280. Which of the following is the recommended state of the bladder during a pelvis exam?

    ___ a.   the bladder should be filled with urine
    ___ b.   the bladder should be emptied just prior to the exam
    ___ c.   the bladder should be filled with contrast
    ___ d.   the bladder should be kept empty via a catheter

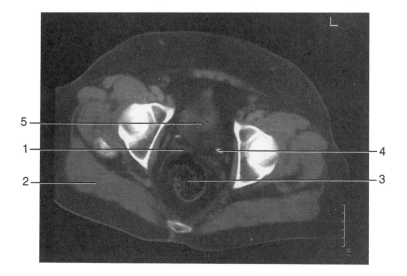

*Figure 22*

281. What number in Figure 22 illustrates a seminal vesicle?

   — a. 1

   — b. 2

   — c. 4

   — d. 5

282. Which of the following is illustrated by #2 in Figure 22?

   — a. erector spinae muscle

   — b. iliacus muscle

   — c. gluteus maximus muscle

   — d. psoas major muscle

283. What anatomical structure is illustrated by #3 in Figure 22?

   — a. prostrate gland

   — b. rectum

   — c. urinary bladder

   — d. uterus

284. What names are used to describe the region below the pelvic brim?

    1. true peivis
    2. lesser pelvis
    3. greater pelvis

    ___ a.  1 and 2
    ___ b.  1 and 3
    ___ c.  2 and 3
    ___ d.  1, 2, & 3

285. What condition is produced when the linea alba is disrupted and fat and bowel penetrate anteriorly through the defect?

    1. inguinal hernia
    2. ventral hernia
    3. intraperitoneal abscess

    ___ a.  1 only
    ___ b.  2 only
    ___ c.  3 only
    ___ d.  1, 2, & 3

286. Which of the following anatomical structures would be visualized first when sagittal reformations are obtained from right to left?

    ___ a.  rectum
    ___ b.  sigmoid colon
    ___ c.  descending colon
    ___ d.  ascending colon

287. What is the primary clinical role of computed tomography for examination of the pelvis when cancer of the urinary bladder is suspected?

    ___ a.  to determine the presence of invasion into the perivesicle fat, adjacent viscera, and pelvic lymph nodes
    ___ b.  to detect microscopic invasion of perivesicle fat
    ___ c.  to be used as a screening procedure for suspected cancer of the urinary bladder
    ___ d.  to determine superficial lesions from one another

288. Which of the following percentages of iodinated contrast media would provide the best diagnostic results if introduced via Foley catheter into the urinary bladder?

   ___ a.  20 - 30%

   ___ b.  40 - 50%

   ___ c.  60- 70%

   ___ d.  80 - 90%

289. Which of the following are indications for CT scanning of the pelvis?

   1.  localization of lesions for radiation therapy planning
   2.  determining the stage of prostate neoplasms
   3.  evaluating the response of disease to chemotherapy

   ___ a.  1 only

   ___ b.  2 only

   ___ c.  3 only

   ___ d.  1, 2, & 3

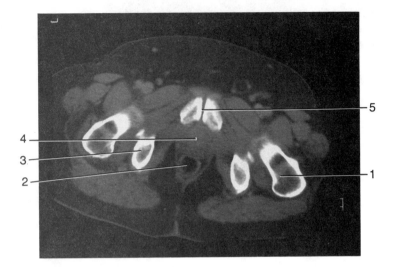

*Figure 23*

290. Which of the following is illustrated by #4 in Figure 23?

___ a. urinary bladder

___ b. prostate gland

___ c. rectum

___ d. seminal vesicle

291. Which of the following is illustrated by #3 in Figure 23?

___ a. ilium

___ b. ischium

___ c. acetabulum

___ d. greater trochanter

292. Which of the following is illustrated by #2 in Figure 23?

___ a. prostate gland

___ b. urinary bladder

___ c. rectum

___ d. sigmoid colon

293. What type of scoutview is recommended for a routine CT examination of the pelvis?

___ a. AP

___ b. lateral

___ c. decubitus

___ d. oblique

294. What type of artifact may be caused by a biopsy needle when performing a biopsy of a lesion located in the pelvis?

___ a. ring artifact

___ b. sampling artifact

___ c. edge gradient artifact

___ d. out of field artifact

295. Which of the following is located between the uterus and rectum?

1. vesicouterine pouch
2. uterovesical pouch
3. rectouterine pouch

___ a. 1 only

___ b. 2 only

___ c. 3 only

___ d. 1, 2, & 3

296. What is the total volume of a pelvis scanned utilizing the helical/spiral acquisition method if the scan time is 1 sec/rotation, total scanning time is 20 seconds, section thickness is 10mm, and tabletop speed is 10mm/sec?

___ a. 100mm

___ b. 200mm

___ c. 300mm

___ d. 400mm

297. Which of the following could make visualization of an undescended testicle in the upper pelvis difficult?

    1.    unopacified bowel loops

    2.    vascular structures

    3.    lymph nodes

    ___  a.  1 and 2

    ___  b.  1 and 3

    ___  c.  2 and 3

    ___  d.  1, 2, & 3

298. Which of the following windowing techniques would provide the best information when a suspected intrapelvic soft tissue mass has invaded the bony pelvis?

    1.    350 window width, 50 window level

    2.    2000 window width, 200 window level

    3.    2000 window width, -200 window level

    ___  a.  1 and 2

    ___  b.  1 and 3

    ___  c.  2 and 3

    ___  d.  1, 2, & 3

299. Which of the following can occur if the technologist selects too low of an mAs value when scanning the pelvis?

    1.    low contrast detectability increases

    2.    low contrast detectability decreases

    3.    loss of detail

    ___  a.  1 and 2

    ___  b.  1 and 3

    ___  c.  2 and 3

    ___  d.  1, 2, & 3

300. Which of the following can occur if a patient is not properly centered for CT examination of the pelvis?

1. out of field artifacts
2. inaccuracy of CT numbers
3. decreased matrix size

___ a. 1 and 2

___ b. 1 and 3

___ c. 2 and 3

___ d. 1, 2, & 3

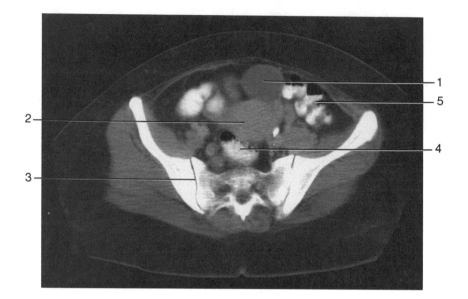

*Figure 24*

301. What is most likely represented by #1 in Figure 24 if the structure has a CT number that equals 0?

    __ a. solid mass

    __ b. cyst

    __ c. acute hematoma

    __ d. calcification

302. Which of the following is illustrated by #3 in Figure 24?

    __ a. acetabulum

    __ b. sacroiliac joint

    __ c. longitudinal fracture

    __ d. iliosacral ligament

303. Which of the following is illustrated by #2 in Figure 24?

  ___ a.   uterus

  ___ b.   urinary bladder

  ___ c.   transverse colon

  ___ d.   rectum

# Musculoskeletal                                    (#304-315)

304. Which of the following scout views should be obtained for CT of the acetabulum?

1.  AP
2.  lateral
3.  oblique

  ___ a.   1 only

  ___ b.   2 only

  ___ c.   3 only

  ___ d.   1, 2, & 3

305. Which of the following are reasons that CT would be the imaging modality of choice when imaging trauma to any part of the musculoskeletal system?

1.  minimal positioning maneuvers are required
2.  complex fractures can be thoroughly defined
3.  manipulation of acquired data allows the evaluation of the extent of soft tissue and bony injuries

  ___ a.   1 and 2

  ___ b.   1 and 3

  ___ c.   2 and 3

  ___ d.   1, 2, & 3

306. Which of the following positions is the patient placed when performing a CT examination of the shoulder and scapula?

  ___ a.   supine with the hands pronated

  ___ b.   supine with the hands supinated

  ___ c.   supine with hands in neutral position

  ___ d.   prone with the hands in neutral position

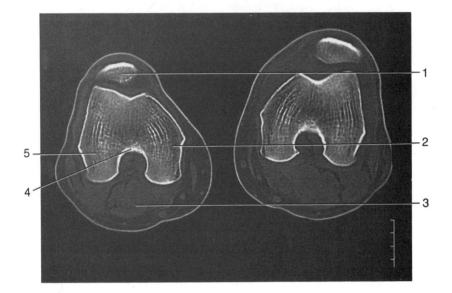

*Figure 25*

307. Which of the following numbers illustrates the intercondylar fossa in Figure 25?

    __ a. 1

    __ b. 2

    __ c. 4

    __ d. 5

308. Which of the following is illustrated by #3 in Figure 25?

    __ a. biceps femoris muscle

    __ b. patellar ligament

    __ c. gastrocnemius muscle

    __ d. popliteal ligament

309. Which of the following is illustrated by #5 in Figure 25?

___ a. lateral condyle of the femur

___ b. medial condyle of the femur

___ c. trochlea

___ d. capitulum

310. Which of the following are requirements for 3D reconstruction when abnormalities are detected by any initial screening examination of the musculoskeletal system?

1. patient immobilization to eliminate motion

2. contiguous non-overlapping sections of the area of interest

3. thin overlapping sections of the area of interest

___ a. 1 and 2

___ b. 1 and 3

___ c. 2 and 3

___ d. 1, 2, & 3

311. Which of the following is true regarding CT of an upper extremity when a soft tissue mass is located on an initial screening scan?

1. a second scan utilizing 8-10mm sections should be obtained through the area of interest

2. contrast media should be introduced in a vein distal to the lesion

3. the scan should include both upper extremities symmetrically positioned

___ a. 1 and 2

___ b. 1 and 3

___ c. 2 and 3

___ d. 1, 2, & 3

312. Which of the following statements is/are true regarding computed tomography compared to other modalities for imaging of the musculoskeletal system?

    1.    computed tomography is superior to angiography when evaluating vascular relationships with soft tissue structures and lesions

    2.    computed tomography is superior to nuclear medicine bone scans for determination of soft tissue position to bone

    3.    computed tomography is superior to conventional radiography for evaluation the extent of intraarticular fracture fragments

    __  a.  1 only

    __  b.  2 only

    __  c.  3 only

    __  d.  1, 2, & 3

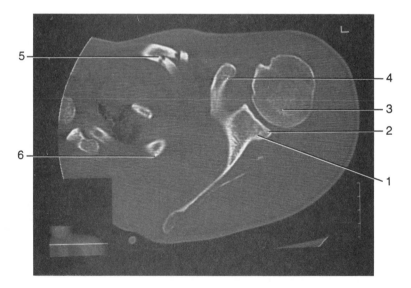

*Figure 26*

313. Which of the following is illustrated by #4 in Figure 26?

    __  a.  acromion process

    __  b.  coracoid process

    __  c.  glenoid

    __  d.  clavicle

314. Which of the following is illustrated by #1 in Figure 26?

    __ a. acromion process

    __ b. coracoid process

    __ c. glenoid

    __ d. clavicle

315. Which of the following is illustrated by #5 in Figure 26?

    __ a. acromion process

    __ b. coracoid process

    __ c. glenoid

    __ d. clavicle

# Physics and Instrumentation    (#316 - 450)

## System Operation & Components    *(#316 - 342)*

316. What type of gas is commonly used in gas-filled computed tomography ionization chamber detectors?

    ___ a.  oxygen

    ___ b.  helium

    ___ c.  neon

    ___ d.  xenon

317. What is the efficiency range of solid state crystal detectors?

    ___ a.  50 - 60%

    ___ b.  70 - 80%

    ___ c.  85 - 89%

    ___ d.  95 - 99%

318. Third generation (rotate/rotate) scanners overcame which of the following limitations?

    ___ a.  detector signal drift sensitivity

    ___ b.  translation motion

    ___ c.  spurious signals from moving signal wires

    ___ d.  cost

319. Which of the following are fundamental considerations in computed tomography x-ray tube life?

    1.  output level
    2.  anode heat load design
    3.  distance from cathode to anode

    ___ a.  1 and 2

    ___ b.  1 and 3

    ___ c.  2 and 3

    ___ d.  1, 2, & 3

320. Which of the following are true when an analog signal is digitized?

1. information is lost
2. the data cannot be returned to an analog state
3. the resulting information cannot be handled by a computer processing system

___ a. 1 only

___ b. 2 only

___ c. 3 only

___ d. 1, 2, & 3

321. Which of the following are capable of storing computed tomography data?

1. optical disk
2. optical tape
3. magnetic tape

___ a. 1 and 2

___ b. 1 and 3

___ c. 2 and 3

___ d. 1, 2, & 3

322. Which of the following are TRUE regarding solid state scintillation detectors?

1. they have better absorption efficiency than xenon detectors
2. they are the only type of detector that can be used in a fourth generation system with changing tube to detector alignment
3. they have poor scatter rejection abilities

___ a. 1 only

___ b. 2 only

___ c. 3 only

___ d. 1, 2, & 3

323. Which of the following are in motion during an exposure with a helical or spiral computed tomography unit?

    1. table
    2. body part of interest
    3. x-ray tube

        __ a.  1 and 2
        __ b.  1 and 3
        __ c.  2 and 3
        __ d.  1, 2, & 3

324. What helical or spiral computed tomography term is defined as: the table increment in distance per mm per 360° gantry rotation divided by the section thickness in mm?

        __ a.  rotation
        __ b.  spiral
        __ c.  helix
        __ d.  pitch

325. What term is used to describe a scanner configuration comprising a 360° ring of detectors set to angle out of the path of a 360° x-ray tube rotation?

        __ a.  nutation
        __ b.  fluxuation
        __ c.  stationary rotation
        __ d.  translate and rotate

326. Which of the following will increase the x-ray beam hardening?

    1. kVp level
    2. tissue density
    3. tissue thickness

        __ a.  1 only
        __ b.  2 only
        __ c.  3 only
        __ d.  1, 2, & 3

327. What effect do array processors have on image processing?

    1.  increase display speed
    2.  increase data available for window width
    3.  decrease processing time

    ___ a.  1 and 2
    ___ b.  1 and 3
    ___ c.  2 and 3
    ___ d.  1, 2, & 3

328. Which chemical is no longer used in scintillation CT detectors?

    1.  sodium iodide
    2.  cesium iodide
    3.  calcium fluoride

    ___ a.  1 and 2
    ___ b.  1 and 3
    ___ c.  2 and 3
    ___ d.  1, 2, & 3

329. Which of the following are effective in reducing scatter radia-tion received by the detectors?

    1.  air gap
    2.  fixed grid
    3.  source collimation

    ___ a.  1 and 2
    ___ b.  1 and 3
    ___ c.  2 and 3
    ___ d.  1, 2, & 3

330. What is the bus in a computer system?

    ___ a.  the basic universal system operating language
    ___ b.  the software used to transfer digital information to a display screen
    ___ c.  a conduit for the transfer of information from one component to another
    ___ d.  a method of dividing up calculation functions between the array processors

331. What determines section thickness?

___ a.  scan arc

___ b.  filtration algorithm

___ c.  incident beam collimation

___ d.  detector alignment

332. Which of the following variables does NOT limit dynamic scanning time?

___ a.  interscan delay

___ b.  scan duration

___ c.  tube heat loading capacity

___ d.  patient exposure

333. If a helical or spiral scanner table is moved at 1.5 cm per gantry rotation and a pitch of 1.2, what will be the section thickness?

___ a.  8.5 mm

___ b.  10.5 mm

___ c.  12.5 mm

___ d.  15.5 mm

334. Which of the following is computer memory that cannot be used for data storage because it contains basic operating instructions for the system?

___ a.  ROM

___ b.  RAM

___ c.  CPU

___ d.  CRT

335. Which of the following are proportional to mAs?

1. length of scan time
2. radiation exposure to the patient
3. x-ray tube heating

___ a.  1 and 2

___ b.  1 and 3

___ c.  2 and 3

___ d.  1, 2, & 3

336. Once secondary scatter has been produced, how is it prevented from reaching the detectors?

    1. pre-patient collimation
    2. post-patient collimation
    3. fine slit collimation

        ___ a. 1 only
        ___ b. 2 only
        ___ c. 3 only
        ___ d. 1, 2, & 3

337. Which of the following helical or spiral scanning pitches would produce oversampling?

        ___ a. 0.8
        ___ b. 1.0
        ___ c. 1.2
        ___ d. 2.0

338. Which of the following are input devices to the central processing unit (CPU)?

    1. track ball
    2. laser film printer
    3. keyboard

        ___ a. 1 and 2
        ___ b. 1 and 3
        ___ c. 2 and 3
        ___ d. 1, 2, & 3

339. Which of the following are advantages of helical or spiral computed tomography units?

    1. shorter scan times
    2. single breath hold technique for many procedures eliminates variation from differences in breath holding
    3. less contrast media is required for many procedures

        ___ a. 1 and 2
        ___ b. 1 and 3
        ___ c. 2 and 3
        ___ d. 1, 2, & 3

340. What range of pressure is used in gas-filled computed tomography ionization chamber detectors?

____ a. 1.5 - 2.0 atm

____ b. 5 - 10 atm

____ c. 20 - 25 atm

____ d. 100 - 250 atm

341. Which of the following factors are effected by a decision to use a pulsed or continuous output x-ray tube in a computed tomography unit?

1. scanning speed
2. quality of amplifiers
3. speed of computer acquisition system

____ a. 1 and 2

____ b. 1 and 3

____ c. 2 and 3

____ d. 1, 2, & 3

342. What effect would an array processor failure have on image processing?

____ a. increase image display time

____ b. halt analog to digital conversions

____ c. lengthen detector data acquisition time

____ d. decrease x-ray tube output

# Image Processing & Display      *(#343-390)*

343. Which of the following defines a pixel?

____ a. positive integrated x-ray exposure limitation

____ b. pre-integrated x-ray entrance loading

____ c. picture element

____ d. miniature display

344. What change will occur in the number of detected photons if a section thickness is changed from 5 mm to 10 mm?

____ a. decrease 50%

____ b. decrease 25%

____ c. increase 50%

____ d. increase 100%

345. What term describes the pencil thin x-ray beam that strikes a single detector?

   __ a.  ray

   __ b.  beam

   __ c.  view

   __ d.  projection

346. The reconstructed image has been described more accurately as a stack of frisbees, rather than the common analogy of a stack of bread slices.  The loss of image that occurs at the edge where each section (slice) abuts the next is caused by the relatively large focal spot of the x-ray tube and which of the following?

   1.   edge effect of the collimator
   2.   x-ray scatter
   3.   reconstruction algorithm

   __ a.  1 and 2

   __ b.  1 and 3

   __ c.  2 and 3

   __ d.  1, 2, & 3

347. Three-dimensional surface rendering is accomplished through which of the following?

   __ a.  overprojecting transverse, coronal, and sagittal scans

   __ b.  rendering pixels containing bone densities transparent

   __ c.  drawing a contour line where the bone to soft tissue interface occurs

   __ d.  eliminating surface details

348. Which of the following will magnify the image?

   __ a.  increasing field of view

   __ b.  decreasing field of view

   __ c.  increasing section thickness

   __ d.  decreasing section thickness

349. Which of the following algorithms are analytical?

    1. iterative
    2. Fourier
    3. back-projection

        ___ a. 1 and 2
        ___ b. 1 and 3
        ___ c. 2 and 3
        ___ d. 1, 2, & 3

350. Which of the following are within the typical range for the maximum angle of rotation for a conventional CT scanner?

        ___ a. 80-90°
        ___ b. 120-180°
        ___ c. 250-300°
        ___ d. 450-500°

351. What is the pixel size if the matrix is 512 x 512 and the field of view is 45 cm?

        ___ a. 0.09 mm
        ___ b. 0.9 mm
        ___ c. 11.4 mm
        ___ d. 2,304 cm

352. Which of the following has a negative CT or Hounsfield number?

        ___ a. bone
        ___ b. blood
        ___ c. water
        ___ d. air

353. Which of the following occurs when too large of a displayed field of view is selected?

    1. the viewer's perceptibility of detail is decreased
    2. the amount of tissue that occupies each pixel increases
    3. the amount of tissue that occupies each pixel decreases

        ___ a. 1 and 2
        ___ b. 1 and 3
        ___ c. 2 and 3
        ___ d. 1, 2, & 3

354. What is a kernel?

    ___ a.  a back projected image

    ___ b.  a reconstruction filter

    ___ c.  a type of detector

    ___ d.  a pixel

355. Which of the following is convolution?

    ___ a.  filtered back-projection

    ___ b.  Fourier transform

    ___ c.  iterative filtration

    ___ d.  three-dimensional rendering

356. Which of the following is NOT a commonly used matrix size?

    ___ a.  256 x 256

    ___ b.  320 x 320

    ___ c.  440 x 440

    ___ d.  512 x 512

357. Which of the following determines the maximum number of shades of gray that can be displayed on the CT monitor?

    ___ a.  window level

    ___ b.  window width

    ___ c.  pixel size

    ___ d.  matrix size

358. How many pixels are in a 512 X 512 matrix?

    ___ a.  26,144

    ___ b.  62,144

    ___ c.  262,144

    ___ d.  1,262,144

359. Which of the following are benefits of narrower section thicknesses?

1. reduced partial volume averaging
2. improved spatial resolution
3. decreased scan time

___ a. 1 and 2
___ b. 1 and 3
___ c. 2 and 3
___ d. 1, 2, & 3

360. Which of the following are required for creating diagnostic multiplanar reformatted images from the original scan?

1. stacked contiguous transverse axial scans
2. stacked non-contiguous transverse axial scans
3. gapped transverse axial scans

___ a. 1 only
___ b. 2 only
___ c. 3 only
___ d. 1, 2, & 3

361. Which of the following determines the linear attenuation coefficient for a material?

1. the density of the material being scanned
2. the atomic number of the material being scanned
3. the energy of the incident photons penetrating the material

___ a. 1 and 2
___ b. 1 and 3
___ c. 2 and 3
___ d. 1, 2, & 3

362. Which of the following represents the z-axis of an imaging plane?

___ a. vertical direction
___ b. horizontal direction
___ c. longitudinal direction
___ d. circular direction

363. Which of the following are factors that effect reconstruction speed of an image?

1. the type of reconstruction algorithm selected
2. the selected matrix size
3. the rate of analog to digital conversion of the detected x-ray signal

___ a. 1 and 2

___ b. 1 and 3

___ c. 2 and 3

___ d. 1, 2, & 3

364. Which of the following is the descriptor that is used to express section thickness?

___ a. modular transfer function

___ b. CT number

___ c. section sensitivity profile

___ d. section spatial thickness profile

365. What is the approximate resolving ability of most cathode ray tube (CRT) viewing monitors?

___ a. 1-2 lp/mm

___ b. 5-7 lp/mm

___ c. 12-15 lp/mm

___ d. 25 lp/mm

366. What substance is represented by a CT or Hounsfield number of 0?

___ a. air

___ b. water

___ c. blood

___ d. bone

367. Which of the following is the term used to describe a voxel value that is the average of multiple tissue types contained within the voxel?

___ a. linear attenuation coefficient

___ b. partial volume averaging

___ c. low contrast resolution

___ d. edge gradient averaging

368. Which of the following could cause a CT scanner to fail quality control tests for resolution?

1. detector vibrations
2. increased tube output
3. decreased electronic noise

___ a. 1 only

___ b. 2 only

___ c. 3 only

___ d. 1, 2, & 3

369. Which of the following parameters should the technologist change to compensate for changes made in section thickness and scanning speed if patient dose is not a factor?

___ a. kVp

___ b. mA

___ c. displayed field of view

___ d. focal spot size

370. Which of the following contains the values of x-ray detector response from all views and rays within a scan?

1. convolved data
2. image data
3. raw data

___ a. 1 only

___ b. 2 only

___ c. 3 only

___ d. 1, 2, & 3

371. Which of the following is the central value in a range of gray shades used to display the image?

    __ a. window width

    __ b. window level

    __ c. region of interest

    __ d. dose index

372. Which of the following would result from decreasing section thickness?

  1. increased resolution

  2. decreased voxel size

  3. increased reconstruction time

    __ a. 1 and 2

    __ b. 1 and 3

    __ c. 2 and 3

    __ d. 1, 2, & 3

373. Which of the following is within the CT or Hounsfield unit range for bone?

    __ a. +1,000

    __ b. +50

    __ c. +15

    __ d. -100

374. Which of the following CT numbers would appear as a gray shades when a window width of 300 and a window level of 0 are selected?

    __ a. CT numbers above +300

    __ b. CT numbers between +150 and +300

    __ c. CT numbers between +150 and -150

    __ d. CT numbers below -150

375. Which of the following CT numbers would appear black when a window width of 200 and a window level of +40 is selected?

    __ a. CT numbers below 0

    __ b. CT numbers below -20

    __ c. CT numbers below -40

    __ d. CT numbers below -60

376. Which of the following represents a volume element?

    __ a. vixel

    __ b. voxel

    __ c. volex

    __ d. volelem

377. What is an algorithm?

    __ a. a set of computer instructions for quality control

    __ b. the scanning parameters

    __ c. a series of mathematical calculations

    __ d. the method used by the detector to send information to the computer for processing

378. Which of the following occur when using a smaller field of view?

    1. each voxel represents less tissue

    2. spatial resolution is increased

    3. display image is magnified

    __ a. 1 and 2

    __ b. 1 and 3

    __ c. 2 and 3

    __ d. 1, 2, & 3

379. Why are laser cameras considered to be superior to multiformat cameras?

    1. laser cameras produce higher contrast film images

    2. laser cameras have no focusing problems

    3. laser cameras are cheaper

    __ a. 1 and 2

    __ b. 1 and 3

    __ c. 2 and 3

    __ d. 1, 2, & 3

380. What determines the intensity of the laser beam in a laser camera?

    __ a. the pixel values in the image data

    __ b. the size of the formatted film region

    __ c. the size of the laser camera

    __ d. the amount of analog information that must be scanned

381. What is the most common of type of film used to record CT examinations?

    __ a. single emulsion

    __ b. double emulsion

    __ c. triple emulsion

    __ d. rare earth

382. What is the voxel size when a CT scan is made with a 5mm section thickness and a 0.75mm pixel size?

    __ a. $1.25mm^3$

    __ b. $2.81mm^3$

    __ c. $3.75mm^3$

    __ d. $4.81mm^3$

383. What substances are represented by CT or Hounsfield numbers above 0?

1. water
2. blood
3. muscle

    __ a. 1 and 2

    __ b. 1 and 3

    __ c. 2 and 3

    __ d. 1, 2, & 3

384. Which of the following information can be derived from a region of interest measurement?

1. mean attenuation values within the region of interest
2. amount of CT number variation within the region of interest
3. standard deviation of attenuation values within the region of interest

___ a. 1 and 2

___ b. 1 and 3

___ c. 2 and 3

___ d. 1, 2, & 3

385. Which of the following provides a graphic presentation of the distribution of CT numbers and the amplitudes of the relative number of points within a particular region of interest?

___ a. Fourier transformation

___ b. linear transfer function

___ c. histogram

___ d. index

386. Which of the following allows helical or spiral data to be changed to planar or axial type data?

___ a. linear transformation

___ b. linear reformation

___ c. linear interpolation

___ d. planar modulation

387. Which of the following are causes of CT number variance within a region of interest measurement?

1. volume averaging
2. artifacts
3. mixed attenuated lesions

___ a. 1 and 2

___ b. 1 and 3

___ c. 2 and 3

___ d. 1, 2, & 3

388. Which of the following are terms used to describe specialized reconstructions that are done after the initial reconstruction process?

1.  retrospective reconstruction
2.  secondary reconstruction
3.  point by point correction reconstruction

    ___ a.  1 and 2
    ___ b.  1 and 3
    ___ c.  2 and 3
    ___ d.  1, 2, & 3

389. Which of the following is true regarding image magnification in computed tomography?

1.  magnification enlarges the information from one pixel and displays it over several pixels
2.  the magnification process requires the use of image data only
3.  the greater the magnification factor used, the better the quality of the image compared to a targeted reconstructed image

    ___ a.  1 and 2
    ___ b.  1 and 3
    ___ c.  2 and 3
    ___ d.  1, 2, & 3

390. Which of the following contribute to interscan delay for section by section conventional CT scanning?

1.  start-stop action of the tube and detector assembly
2.  start-stop action necessary for patient breathing
3.  table indexing

    ___ a.  1 and 2
    ___ b.  1 and 3
    ___ c.  2 and 3
    ___ d.  1, 2, & 3

# Image Quality                                      *(#391-423)*

391. Which of the following increase signal to noise ratio?

1.  increased mAs
2.  wider section thickness
3.  increased detection efficiency

___ a.  1 and 2

___ b.  1 and 3

___ c.  2 and 3

___ d.  1, 2, & 3

392. What is an appropriate compensation to avoid quantum noise when performing thin section computed tomography?

___ a.  increase mAs

___ b.  decrease field of view

___ c.  increase matrix size

___ d.  decrease scan speed

393. Which of the following increases spatial resolution?

1.  increase focal spot size
2.  increase matrix size
3.  decrease the number of projections obtained

___ a.  1 only

___ b.  2 only

___ c.  3 only

___ d.  1, 2, & 3

394. Which of the following refers to the relationship of CT numbers to the linear attenuation coefficients of the imaged object?

___ a.  contrast resolution

___ b.  spatial resolution

___ c.  linearity

___ d.  clarity

395. Which of the following accurately describes the relationship between section thickness and noise?

    __ a.  if section thickness increases, noise increases

    __ b.  if section thickness increases, noise decreases

    __ c.  if section thickness decreases, noise decreases

    __ d.  if section thickness decreases, noise remains unchanged

396. Which of the following are types of noise?

    1.    quantum noise
    2.    structural noise
    3.    electronic noise

    __ a.  1 and 2

    __ b.  1 and 3

    __ c.  2 and 3

    __ d.  1, 2, & 3

397. Which of the following results from applying a high spatial frequency or high pass filter to the reconstruction process of an abdominal scan?

    1.    increase in contrast resolution
    2.    increase in image noise
    3.    increase in edge enhancement

    __ a.  1 and 2

    __ b.  1 and 3

    __ c.  2 and 3

    __ d.  1, 2, & 3

398. What term is used to describe as the ability to display an image of a large object that is only slightly different in density from its surroundings?

    __ a.  spatial resolution

    __ b.  contrast resolution

    __ c.  linearity

    __ d.  clarity

399. Which of the following is true regarding image quality of computed tomography compared to conventional screen-film radiography image quality?

   1. CT contrast resolution is significantly superior than that of conventional radiography

   2. CT spatial resolution is significantly superior than that of conventional radiography

   3. CT can detect density differences of 0.25%-0.5% compared to 10% for conventional radiography

      __ a. 1 and 2
      __ b. 1 and 3
      __ c. 2 and 3
      __ d. 1, 2, & 3

400. What object size can be resolved if a CT scanner has a limiting resolution of 8 lp/cm?

      __ a. 0.3mm
      __ b. 0.6mm
      __ c. 1.25mm
      __ d. 3.75mm

401. Which of the following image characteristics can be obtained from a CT number water calibration test?

   1. high contrast resolution
   2. spatial uniformity
   3. noise

      __ a. 1 and 2
      __ b. 1 and 3
      __ c. 2 and 3
      __ d. 1, 2, & 3

402. What is the acceptable range of CT numbers that determines the success or failure of a scanner for the water calibration test which is done by imaging a cylindrical water filled phantom

with a mid phantom ROI measurement that includes 200-300 pixels?

___ a.   -3 to +3 HU from the attenuation value of water

___ b.   -6 to +6 HU from the attenuation value of water

___ c.   -10 to +10 HU from the attenuation value of water

___ d.   -20 to +20 HU from the attenuation value of water

403. Spatial resolution refers to resolution coordinates in which imaging planes?

1.   x
2.   y
3.   z

___ a.   1 and 2
___ b.   1 and 3
___ c.   2 and 3
___ d.   1, 2, & 3

404. Which of the following should be viewed with relatively wide window widths?

1.   lung
2.   inner ear
3.   brain

___ a.   1 and 2
___ b.   1 and 3
___ c.   2 and 3
___ d.   1, 2, & 3

405. Quantum noise is decreased by which of the following?

1.   decreasing mAs
2.   decreasing kVp
3.   increasing section thickness

___ a.   1 only
___ b.   2 only
___ c.   3 only
___ d.   1, 2, & 3

406. How often should an average CT number water calibration test be performed?

___ a. daily

___ b. weekly

___ c. monthly

___ d. yearly

407. Which of the following accurately describes the relationship between patient dose and pitch?

___ a. if pitch increases, patient dose increases

___ b. if pitch increases, patient dose decreases

___ c. if pitch decreases, patient dose decreases

___ d. if pitch decreases, patient dose remains unchanged

408. What does the convolution process do to enhance image quality when it is added to the back projection reconstruction process?

___ a. changes the linear attenuation coefficient values eliminating unwanted structures from the image

___ b. increases the number of samples measured at the detector eliminating ailiasing artifacts

___ c. changes the shape of the attenuation profiles eliminating streak and star artifacts

___ d. increases the matrix size eliminating partial volume artifacts

409. Which of the following is defined as the ability to distinguish details in objects of different densities a small distance apart?

___ a. contrast resolution

___ b. cross field uniformity

___ c. spatial resolution

___ d. interpolation

410. What is a term that is used to describe contrast resolution?

___ a. high spatial detectibility

___ b. high contrast detectibility

___ c. low spatial detectibility

___ d. low contrast detectibility

411. Which of the following would maximize soft tissue resolution?

    1.    low spatial frequency or low pass algorithm

    2.    narrow window widths

    3.    low window levels

    __ a.   1 and 2

    __ b.   1 and 3

    __ c.   2 and 3

    __ d.   1, 2, & 3

412. What is the primary type of interaction that contributes to the subject contrast in CT images?

    __ a.   pair production

    __ b.   photoelectric effect

    __ c.   Compton scattering

    __ d.   linear attenuation

413. Which of the following is the most commonly used descriptor for quantifying spatial resolution?

    __ a.   modular transfer function

    __ b.   multiple scan average dose

    __ c.   computed tomography dose index

    __ d.   multi energy spatial registration

414. Which of the following accurately describes the relationship between radiation dose and noise?

    __ a.   if radiation dose increases, noise increases

    __ b.   if radiation dose increases, noise decreases

    __ c.   if radiation dose decreases, noise decreases

    __ d.   if radiation dose decreases, noise remains unchanged

415. Which of the following is the primary factor that determines the degree of contrast resolution that a CT system is capable of producing?

    __ a.   signal to noise ratio

    __ b.   spatial to noise ratio

    __ c.   frequency to noise ratio

    __ d.   attenuation to noise ratio

416. Which of the following would result in a decrease of low contrast resolution?

    1. application of a low spatial frequency algorithm to a CT scan of the abdomen

    2. decrease in the number of photons at the detector

    3. decrease patient dose

    ___ a. 1 and 2

    ___ b. 1 and 3

    ___ c. 2 and 3

    ___ d. 1, 2, & 3

417. Which of the following will double the number of detected x-ray photons if kVp, mA, and time remain constant?

    ___ a. increase section thickness from 5mm to 10mm

    ___ b. increase section thickness from 1mm to 3mm

    ___ c. decrease section thickness from 10mm to 5mm

    ___ d. decrease section thickness from 3mm to 1mm

418. Which of the following is responsible for an increase in quantum noise for a dynamic CT scan sequence?

    ___ a. decrease in technical factors necessary to perform a dynamic sequence

    ___ b. increase in technical factors necessary to perform a dynamic sequence

    ___ c. increase in the speed of the data samples reaching the detectors

    ___ d. decreases in the speed of the data samples reaching the detectors

419. Which of the following determines a CT scanners performance relative to a low contrast resolution test pattern?

    ___ a. the size of the row of holes in which all holes can be clearly visualized

    ___ b. the distance between the rows of holes in which all holes can be clearly visualized

    ___ c. the shape distortion between the rows of holes in which all holes can be clearly visualized

    ___ d. the width of the row of holes in which all holes can be clearly visualized

420. Which of the following maximizes spatial resolution for a CT scan of the temporal bones?

    1.  high spatial frequency algorithm
    2.  thin section thickness
    3.  small FOV

    ___ a.  1 and 2
    ___ b.  1 and 3
    ___ c.  2 and 3
    ___ d.  1, 2, & 3

421. Which of the following are true regarding multiple scan average dose (MSAD)?

    1.  MSAD represents an average dose delivered to a patient for a series of scans
    2.  if the scan table index decreases, the MSAD increases
    3.  MSAD represents the dose that the center section receives for a series of scans

    ___ a.  1 and 2
    ___ b.  1 and 3
    ___ c.  2 and 3
    ___ d.  1, 2, & 3

422. Which of the following are true regarding the computed tomography dose index (CTDI)?

    1.  CTDI is the area of one section dose profile divided by the scan section thickness for contiguous sections
    2.  the CTDI of a scanner is measured with an ionization chamber
    3.  the CTDI equals the MSAD if the scan table index equals section thickness

    ___ a.  1 and 2
    ___ b.  1 and 3
    ___ c.  2 and 3
    ___ d.  1, 2, & 3

423. Which of the following comprises an oversampling technique?

    ___ a. shifting the detector 1/2 the distance between the previous section

    ___ b. repeating a filter algorithm to refine the spatial resolution

    ___ c. aligning the central axis of rotation with a point that is 1/4 the width of the detector

    ___ d. combining the data from two scans to create an entirely new perspective

# Artifacts (#424-450)

424. What type of scan geometry is responsible for producing ring artifacts?

    ___ a. translate-rotate

    ___ b. rotate-rotate

    ___ c. rotate only

    ___ d. helical/spiral

425. Which of the following types of artifacts can be caused by unexpected beam hardening due to kVp level, tissue thickness, or tissue density?

1. low density streak adjacent to high density structures
2. general CT number shift
3. cupping artifact

    ___ a. 1 and 2

    ___ b. 1 and 3

    ___ c. 2 and 3

    ___ d. 1, 2, & 3

426. What is the cause for the "cupping" artifact?

    ___ a. the computer overcorrects for beam hardening

    ___ b. the beam encounters metal in the body

    ___ c. the body hardens the beam thus lowering the attenuation numbers in the center

    ___ d. the body hardens the beam thus increasing the attenuation numbers in the center

427. What is the cause for the "capping" artifact?

___ a.  the computer overcorrects for beam hardening

___ b.  the beam encounters metal in the body

___ c.  the body hardens the beam thus lowering the attenuation numbers in the center

___ d.  the body hardens the beam thus increasing the attenuation numbers in the center

428. What is the cause for "star" artifacts?

___ a.  small differences in tissue interfaces

___ b.  large differences in tissue interfaces

___ c.  low density objects in the patient

___ d.  high density objects in the patient

429. What is the primary reason streak artifacts arise from patient motion during a CT scan?

___ a.  inability of the reconstruction algorithm to compensate for the inconsistencies of the voxel attenuations arising from the edge of the moving part

___ b.  inability of low energy photons to reach the part being scanned

___ c.  inability of the tube to stay aligned with the detector array

___ d.  insufficient number of data samples for the spatial frequencies encountered in the body

430. Which of the following can be described as bands or streaks that appear across an area due to bone and soft tissue attenuation values in the same pixel?

___ a.  tube arcing artifacts

___ b.  beam hardening artifacts

___ c.  partial volume artifacts

___ d.  full volume artifacts

431. Which of the following influences a scanners ability to image metallic objects in the body with a reduction of artifacts?

    __ a. detector arrays dynamic range

    __ b. detector to tube alignment

    __ c. rotational speed of the scanner

    __ d. type of collimation filter used

432. Which of the following will reduce the effects of beam hardening?

    1. employ mathematical corrections to the detector output
    2. added filtration near the x-ray tube
    3. increase scan field of view

    __ a. 1 and 2

    __ b. 1 and 3

    __ c. 2 and 3

    __ d. 1, 2, & 3

433. Which of the following is a streak artifact oriented tangentially to a flat surface having a high spatial frequency?

    __ a. low contrast artifact

    __ b. edge gradient artifact

    __ c. equipment induced artifact

    __ d. signal artifact

434. Which of the following would minimize the effect of partial volume artifacts while maintaining the same signal to noise performance?

    1. decrease section thickness
    2. increase the mAs
    3. increase pixel size

    __ a. 1 and 2

    __ b. 1 and 3

    __ c. 2 and 3

    __ d. 1, 2, & 3

435. Which of the following allows an increase in scan time to reduce motion artifacts for fourth generation scanners?

___ a.  if the increase is used to perform a half scan

___ b.  if the increase is used to perform a full scan

___ c.  if the increase is used to perform an underscan

___ d.  if the increase is used to perform an overscan

436. Which of the following cause a beam hardening effect that result in out-of-field artifacts?

1.  thoracotomy tubes
2.  patient's arms
3.  ventilator tubing

___ a.  1 and 2

___ b.  1 and 3

___ c.  2 and 3

___ d.  1, 2, & 3

437. Which of the following effects contribute to the formation of artifacts when structures contain metal such as surgical clips and orthopedic prostheses?

1.  edge gradient effect
2.  nonlinear partial volume effect
3.  beam hardening effect

___ a.  1 and 2

___ b.  1 and 3

___ c.  2 and 3

___ d.  1, 2, & 3

438. Which of the following are functions of a "bow tie" filter?

1.  reduce beam hardening artifacts
2.  reduce scatter radiation
3.  increase x-ray output

___ a.  1 and 2

___ b.  1 and 3

___ c.  2 and 3

___ d.  1, 2, & 3

439. Which of the following algorithms are used to remove streak artifacts that occur from continuous patient transport during helical/spiral CT?

1. iterative algorithm
2. interpolation algorithm
3. filtered back projection algorithm

____ a. 1 only

____ b. 2 only

____ c. 3 only

____ d. 1, 2, & 3

440. Which of the following is produced on a three dimensional reconstructed image if the patient moves during the scanning sequence?

____ a. step-like contours that may resemble fractures

____ b. ring-like artifacts that may resemble large tumors

____ c. out of field artifacts that obscure the anatomy of interest

____ d. star-like artifacts that obscure the anatomy of interest

441. Which of the following can occur on an image due to patient motion?

1. image ghosting
2. image blurring
3. streak artifacts

____ a. 1 and 2

____ b. 1 and 3

____ c. 2 and 3

____ d. 1, 2, & 3

442. What type of artifact is characterized by streaking from high frequency interfaces which result from too few samples or views obtained?

____ a. ailiasing artifact

____ b. gradient field artifact

____ c. spatial artifact

____ d. contrast artifact

443. Which of the following will eliminate ring artifacts?

  ___ a.  increase the scan field of view

  ___ b.  recalibrate the detector gain

  ___ c.  decrease the mAs

  ___ d.  decrease kVp

444. What is the cause of a straight line artifact on third and fourth generation scanograms?

  ___ a.  patient motion

  ___ b.  sample ailiasing

  ___ c.  faulty detector channel

  ___ d.  tube arching

445. What causes an annular ring artifact to be small in diameter?

  ___ a.  one detector out of calibration near the edge of the detector fan array

  ___ b.  one detector out of calibration near the center of the detector fan array

  ___ c.  patient movement near the edge of the detector fan array

  ___ d.  patient movement near the center of the detector fan array

446. Which of the following can cause edge gradient artifacts?

  1.  biopsy needle
  2.  bone to soft tissue interfaces
  3.  cracks in the scanning table

  ___ a.  1 and 2

  ___ b.  1 and 3

  ___ c.  2 and 3

  ___ d.  1, 2, & 3

447. Which of the following will reduce motion artifacts?

1. decrease scan time
2. decrease matrix size
3. decrease displayed field of view

___ a. 1 only

___ b. 2 only

___ c. 3 only

___ d. 1, 2, & 3

448. Which of the following are directly responsible for creating a tube arching artifact?

1. misalignment of the x-ray tube and detector array
2. vaporization of the anode and filament in an x-ray tube
3. excessive mechanical wear in the motion of the gantry

___ a. 1 only

___ b. 2 only

___ c. 3 only

___ d. 1, 2, & 3

449. Which of the following degrade three dimensional (3D) CT images?

1. missing sections from the selected stack
2. beam hardening artifacts
3. patient motion

___ a. 1 & 2

___ b. 1 & 3

___ c. 2 & 3

___ d. 1, 2, & 3

450. Which of the following reduces artifacts from scatter radiation?

1. post patient collimation
2. secondary detectors placed outside the reach of primary radiation
3. narrow window widths

___ a. 1 and 2

___ b. 1 and 3

___ c. 2 and 3

___ d. 1, 2, & 3

# Patient Care (#1-90)

## Patient Preparation (#1-12)

1. **(D)** Proper informed consent is synonymous with full disclosure. Proper informed consent requires full disclosure of the procedure and the technique involved for completing the specific exam. Disclosure of the risks, benefits, and alternatives is essential to receiving legal consent from a patient. **informed consent, ethics (Torres, Adler, Ehrlich)**

2. **(D)** The patient's medical record includes all documents regarding the patient that are collected. This includes records of medications given, consent forms, and radiographs. **medical record (Torres, Adler, Ehrlich)**

3. **(D)** Although no method should be used by itself, questioning the patient, reading the wrist identification band, and checking the bed name plate are all valid cross-checks of patient identification. **patient identification (Torres, Adler, Ehrlich)**

4. **(C)** Respondeat superior ("let the master answer") holds that the employer is responsible for the acts of the radiographer. **malpractice (Tortorici, Adler, Torres)**

5. **(B)** Minors and persons who have had their civil rights removed (such as prisoners) may undergo procedures upon the consent of their guardian. In the case of a prisoner, this is often the officer in charge of the prisoner. Beyond being a minor, the age of a patient is not a determinant in consent. **informed consent (Torres, Adler, Ehrlich)**

6. **(D)** A radiographer is responsible to provide the physician with all information relative to radiologic diagnosis according to the *Principals of Professional Conduct* of the American Registry of Radiologic Technologists. This case clearly involves providing additional information from the patient history to the physician before

proceeding with the examination. **code of ethics, ethics (Torres, Adler, Ehrlich)**

7. **(B)** When a patient denies knowledge of the possible effects of the use on contrast media, the effects should be explained and verification of understanding, preferably in writing, should be obtained from the patient. **consent (Torres, Adler, Ehrlich)**

8. **(A)** If contrast agents are to be used or the procedure involves an interventional technique, the patient is usually required to complete a consent form. **consent form (Snopek, Ballinger, Berland)**

9. **(D)** Correct patient positioning, proper breathing instructions, and proper selection of technical factors should be carried out by the technologist before any exam begins. **technologist responsibilities ( Adler, Torres, Berland)**

10. **(D)** Patient positioning is determined by the desired plane of anatomy that is to be imaged, the patients' ability to cooperate, the limitation of the gantry angulation and the diameter of the opening for the patient into the gantry. **scanning procedure (Berland, Ballinger)**

11. **(A)** Any movement during the examination is undesirable and can lead to a loss of diagnostic information. **scanning procedure (Ballinger, Berland, Adler)**

12. **(D)** Patient's allergies, cardiac history, and renal history should all be checked prior to beginning any examination requiring the introduction of contrast media to a patient. **contrast media (Torres, Adler, Ehrlich)**

## Assessment and Monitoring *(#13-30)*

13. **(B)** The normal diastolic pressure ranges from 60 - 80 mm HG and normal systolic pressure ranges from 110 - 140mm HG. **blood pressure, vital signs (Torres, Adler, Ehrlich)**

14. **(D)** The average pulse rate of an infant is 115 - 130 beats per minute. **vital signs, pulse (Torres, Adler, Ehrlich)**

15. **(A)** A patient in insulin shock who is still conscious requires something with sugar. **diabetic emergencies (Torres, Adler, Ehrlich)**

16. **(C)** Hypoxia describes a state of oxygen deficiency at the tissue level. **hypoxia, oxygen (Torres, Adler, Ehrlich)**

17. **(B)** Syncope is a transient loss of consciousness due to inadequate blood flow to the brain. **syncope (Torres, Adler, Ehrlich)**

18. **(B)** The average range of rate of respiration (one inspiration and one expiration) for an adult is 10 - 20 respirations/min. **vital signs, respiration (Torres, Adler, Ehrlich)**

19. **(A)** A nonrebreathing mask provides the highest oxygen concentration. **respiration, oxygen therapy (Torres, Adler)**

20. **(B)** Dyspnea is air hunger resulting in labored or difficult breathing sometimes accompanied by pain. **respiration, dyspnea (Torres, Adler)**

21. **(D)** If you suspect that your patient has had respiratory or cardiac arrest,the first consideration is an open airway. Next, rescue breathing by means of the mouth-to-mouth technique provides adequate oxygen to support if the patient's lungs are adequately inflated and then external cardiac compression to provide circulation of blood. **respiratory failure (Torres, Adler, Ehrlich)**

22. **(B)** The human brain can survive without oxygen for about only four minutes. **respiration, cardiopulmonary resuscitation (Torres, Adler, Ehrlich)**

23. **(B)** Direct pressure should be applied to a wound that is bleeding profusely. **emergency care (Torres, Adler, Ehrlich)**

24. **(D)** Hypovolemic shock is caused by an excessive loss of blood. **shock (Torres, Adler, Ehrlich)**

25. **(B)** If a diabetic patient has taken his normal dose of insulin but has been NPO since midnight there is a

chance the patient will develop insulin shock. **diabetes mellitus (Torres, Adler, Ehrlich)**

26. **(D)** Nitroglycerin is a rapid acting vasodilator that reduces vascular resistance and lower blood pressure. **vasodilators (Torres, Adler)**

27. **(C)** PTT represents partial thromboplastin time. **normal laboratory values (Mosby's, Dorland's)**

28. **(A)** The normal range for a PTT coagulation study in 20 - 37 seconds. **normal laboratory values (Mosby's, Fischbach)**

29. **(A)** The normal range for a (PT) prothrombin time coagulation study is 10 - 14 seconds. The theraputic range for oral anticoagulant therapy is 2 - 2.5 times the normal limit. **normal laboratory values (Mosby's, Fischbach)**

30. **(A)** Average adult BUN range is from 2.9 - 8.9 mmol/L or around 5-20 mg/d. **normal laboratory values (Mosby's, Dorland's)**

# IV Procedures                    *(#31-54)*

31. **(D)** An autoclave sterilizes by steam pressure, usually at about 250 degrees F. **sterilization technique (Torres, Adler)**

32. **(D)** In enteric isolation, the infective agent resides in the gastrointestinal tract and its product, feces. **isolation procedure (Torres, Adler)**

33. **(B)** Medical asepsis is the process of reducing the probability of infectious organisms being transmitted to someone who is susceptible. **infection control (Torres, Ehrlich, Adler)**

34. **(C)** When the sterilization of an object is in question, it must be discarded. **sterilization (Torres, Adler, Ehrlich)**

35. **(C)** Infection proceeds from incubation to prodromal to full active to convalescent infection. **infection (Torres, Ehrlich, Adler)**

36. **(C)** Microorganisms that are capable of forming spores can survive high heat, chemicals, dry periods, etc., and remain viable when favorable conditions are available. **infection control (Torres, Ehrlich, Adler)**

37. **(A)** Disinfection involves the destruction of pathogens by using chemicals. **infection control (Torres, Ehrlich, Adler)**

38. **(B)** Steam under pressure is the most effective and convenient method of sterilization for items that can withstand high temperatures. **sterilization (Ehrlich, Torres, Adler)**

39. **(A)** Nosocomial infections are those that are acquired by a patient while in a health-care institution. **infection control (Torres, Ehrlich, Adler)**

40. **(B)** 18 - 20-gauge butterfly needles, 1 inch in length are the most commonly used butterfly needles in the diagnostic imaging department. **intravenous infusions (Torres, Adler)**

41. **(A)** A parenteral route is any means that bypasses the digestive tract. **parenteral route (Torres, Adler)**

42. **(C)** The patient is to be observed following medication administration for at least 30 minutes. **intravenous administration (Torres, Adler)**

43. **(A)** A venous catheter, also called angiocatheter, is a plastic tubing with a needle through the tubing for insertion into the vein. Once the needle is in the vein, the catheter is moved into place within the vein and the needle removed. **intravenous infusions (Torres, Adler)**

44. **(B)** The antecubital or medial (basilic) vein is preferred because the lateral vein may lead into a cephalic vein, which tends to occlude when the arms are raised. **vascular contrast (Adler, Torres)**

45. **(C)** An intradermal injection is an injection made between the layers of the skin. **parenteral route (Torres, Adler)**

46. **(B)** The antecubital or medial (basilic) vein is preferred because the lateral vein may lead into a cephalic vein,

which tends to occlude when the arms are raised. **vascular contrast (Adler, Torres)**

47. **(A)** For prolonged IV infusions, veins in the forearm and the back of the hand are preferred. **intravenous infusions (Torres, Adler)**

48. **(D)** Hypertonic solutions, those to be administered rapidly, and viscid (thick and sticky) solutions should be administered into a large vein in the forearm. **intravenous infusions (Torres, Adler)**

49. **(C)** For a single scan sequence, 100 to 180 ml of 60% iodinated contrast medium may be given. **contrast dose (Berland, Morgan)**

50. **(A)** The delay after initiating scanning may be only about 10-20 seconds for the chest. **contrast dose (Berland, Morgan)**

51. **(B)** The delay after initiating scanning may be approximately 30 - 45 seconds for the liver. **contrast dose (Berland, Haaga, Lee, Lee)**

52. **(B)** A 30 - 45 second delay is used for the liver because of the desire to obtain scans only after contrast material reaches the portal vein. The exact delay also depends on the scanning method and type of scanner used. **contrast dose (Berland, Lee, Haaga)**

53. **(A)** Patients having a brain scan without using any type of contrast media do not need any type of preparation. **contrast dose (Berland, Ballinger, Morgan)**

54. **(B)** The delay after initiating scanning may be only about 20 - 30 seconds for the pancreas. **contrast dose (Berland, Lee)**

55. **(C)** Higher iodine concentration results in increased contrast media viscosity making injection more difficult. **contrast media (Ballinger, Snopek)**

56. **(C)** A patient who is well hydrated is less likely to experience renal failure following an ionic contrast injection. **contrast media (Torres, Adler)**

57. **(A)** Ionic contrast media dissociate into two charged particles one positive and one negative for every three iodine

molecules present. The average osmolarity of blood is 300 mosm/kg compared to 1400-1600 mosm\kg of iodinated contrast media therefore, ionic contrast media is a hyperosmolar solution. Ionic contrast media used in CT is water soluble. **contrast media, iodinated contrast agents (Torres, Adler, Ehrlich)**

58. **(B)** The absorption of primary photons causes positive contrast material to produce an area of reduced image density. **contrast material (Torres, Adler)**

59. **(D)** Headaches, aphasia, and unconsciousness are all possible adverse effects when injecting contrast media. **adverse effects, contrast material (Torres, Adler, Ehrlich)**

60. **(C)** A vasodilator will relax vascular walls to permit greater blood flow. **drugs (Torres, Adler)**

61. **(B)** Barium sulfate is used for visualization of the gastrointestinal tract when a perforation is not suspected. Barium sulfite is extremely toxic and is never used for radiologic imaging. **barium studies (Torres, Adler)**

62. **(B)** A bismuth laxative is partially radiopaque and will produce artifacts after it coats the intestine. Castor oil, saline enemas, and soap suds enemas are all acceptable cleansing methods. **cathartics, laxatives (Ehrlich, Torres, Adler)**

63. **(C)** When scanning for gynecologic malignancies and bladder and prostate carcinoma about 300 - 500 ml of rectal contrast should be given to patients capable of tolerating it. **pelvis studies (Berland, Morgan)**

64. **(B)** Warming contrast material decreases its viscosity. **contrast material, automatic injectors (Torres, Snopek, Adler)**

65. **(D)** Histamine is a bronchial and tracheal smooth muscle constrictor and it induces capillary dilation which is believed to cause extravasation into the surrounding tissues producing hives. Excessive histamine release causes a decrease in blood pressure. **histamine (Torres, Adler, Ehrlich, Porth)**

66. **(C)** If patients are unable to ingest oral contrast, it may be injected through a nasogastric tube. **oral contrast (Berland, Morgan)**

67. **(A)** Parenteral denotes any route other than the alimentary canal, such as intravenous, subcutaneous, intramuscular or mucosal. **injections (Torres, Adler, Ehrlich)**

68. **(B)** An IV solution should be kept between 18 to 20 inches above the patient at all times. **injections (Torres, Adler, Ehrlich)**

69. **(B)** A safe rule to follow is to allow the solution to infuse at 15 - 20 drops/min. **intravenous infusions (Torres, Adler, Ehrlich)**

70. **(D)** Grastrografin (Winthrop)and Gastroview (Mallinckrodt, Inc.) are water-soluble oral contrast agents. **contrast media (Berland, Morgan)**

71. **(A)** Oral contrast (Gastrografin) should be diluted to an approximately a 1 to 3% solution. Mixing 3 ml of 60% contrast solution to 100 ml of water would provide a 3% concentration. **oral contrast (Berland, Morgan)**

72. **(C)** When scanning the upper abdomen, a total of 300 - 1,000 ml of contrast material should be given, depending on the reasons for and the extent of the examination. **oral contrast (Berland, Morgan)**

73. **(C)** Enemas from about 300 - 1000 ml should be given whenever scanning the pelvis. This amount is usually sufficient to opacify the rectosigmoid and portions of the descending colon. **rectal contrast (Berland, Morgan, Bontrager)**

74. **(D)** To aid in easier anatomical localization of the vagina a tampon should routinely be used. Insertion of a tampon produces an entrapment of air. **rectal contrast (Bontrager, Berland, Morgan)**

75. **(C)** Barium sulfate suspensions must be of low concentrations to avoid beam hardening artifacts. Also, delays after ingestion allow water to be absorbed by the bowel which leaves residual barium and also causes beam hardening artifacts. **contrast media (Bontrager, Morgan, Berland)**

76. **(B)** Contrast media viscosity is inversely related to temperature. At higher temperatures, the contrast mate-

rial is less viscous and easier to inject. **automatic injector (Ballinger, Torres, Snopek)**

77. **(C)** Increasing catheter diameter will increase the delivery rate of contrast material. Increases in contrast viscosity, contrast concentration and catheter length will all cause delivery rates to be decreased. **contrast material (Snopek, Ballinger)**

78. **(A)** Iodinated contrast media studies should be performed first, with all examinations performed in the following order of sequence: urinary, biliary, lower gastrointestinal, upper gastrointestinal. **contrast media (Ehrlich, Adler, Torres)**

79. **(C)** If an examination is being performed primarily to study the stomach, the patient is given 350 - 500 ml contrast to drink immediately prior to the study. **oral contrast material (Seeram, Berland)**

80. **(B)** Dynamic incremental CT consists of rapid serial scanning at contiguous levels during a bolus injection of contrast material. This is the preferred technique for examining the liver. It consists of injecting a large amount of contrast material (about 150 - 180 ml) in 2 minutes or less while the entire region is scanned. **contrast material (Seeram, Berland)**

81. **(C)** Injection time is calculated as volume/time so $30/3.7 = 8.1$ seconds. **automatic injectors (Snopek, Ballinger)**

82. **(D)** Most early CT scanners employed a single kVp selection that ranged between 140 and 150. **CT scanners, generations (Berland, Seeram)**

83. **(B)** Compton effect occurs when an incoming x-ray photon strikes a target atom and uses a portion of its energy to eject an outer shell electron. The remainder of the photon's energy proceeds in a different direction than the incoming photon. Most of the occupational worker's exposure to radiation comes from Compton scatter. **Compton effect, scatter (Carlton, Adler)**

84. **(D)** Milliamperage (mA) reading indicates the maximum rate of x-ray output. **milliamperage, x-ray output (Adler, Carlton)**

85. **(B)** Multiple scans at a single level and high resolution scans with long scan times would increase patient radiation exposure. **radiation dose, procedures (Berland, Seeram)**

86. **(B)** The typical skin dose using the manufacturer's suggested mAs and kVp settings for a scanogram is approximately 0.05-0.1 rad. **scanogram, radiation exposure (Berland, Seeram)**

87. **(B)** Lead from shields causes artifacts on the image and the rotational scheme of the x-ray source reduces the effectiveness of shielding a patient during a CT scan. **radiation protection (Seeram, Berland)**

88. **(A)** The first trimester is the most critical period to avoid irradiation of the embryo or fetus. **radiation protection (Carlton, Adler)**

89. **(C)** The MPD for a pregnant women is 0.5 rem. **MPD, radiation protection (Carlton, Adler)**

90. **(B)** Blood forming organs are the most radiosensitive of the structures listed. **radiosensitivity, blood forming organs (Carlton, Adler)**

# Imaging Procedures  *(#91-315)*

## Head                                                    *(#91-135)*

91. **(A)** The lateral scanogram allows calculation of angulation of the gantry. **scout view, scanogram, brain (Berland, Brooker)**

92. **(C)** The angle is 10-20 degrees depending on the specific area of interest. **procedure (Brooker, Lee)**

93. **(C)** Routine section thickness may be up to 10 mm although the area of the posterior fossa may be done somewhat thinner. **brain, procedure (Seeram, Brooker)**

94. **(A)** IV contrast may be used to demonstrate pathologies affecting the blood brain barrier, and positive (iodinated) intrathecal contrast media is utilized to outline certain structures. **procedure, spine (Brooker, Seeram)**

95. **(A)** The supine, head first position is the most comfortable patient position for head studies which allow for individual positioning of the patients head. **procedure, head, preparation (Brooker, Berland, Seeram)**

96. **(A)** The olfactory and optic cranial nerves are the first and second cranial nerves and are located in the first portion of the brain which is called the forebrain. **cranial nerves, forebrain (Porth, Ballinger)**

97. **(D)** Stereotaxis is a procedure combining the use of computed tomography with a stereotactic guidance system for accurate localization of brain lesions, and can be used for surgery,biopsy, and radiation therapy planning procedures. **stereotaxis, computed tomography stereotactic guidance systems (Berland, Haaga)**

98. **(C)** The sharp convolution filter is preferable for imaging high contrast areas such as the temporal bones and is used to increase edge enhancement. **internal auditory canals, convolution filters (Berland, Haaga)**

99. **(D)** Coronal imaging of the orbits is useful in assessing the floor and roof of the orbits and location of foreign bodies

in the orbits. **coronal imaging, orbits (Haaga, Seeram)**

100. **(B)** Two weeks after a stroke occurs, the area of infarction may become isodense with the brain, therefore the infarcted area would have the same attenuation value as normal brain tissue. The introduction of intravenous contrast material is necessary to visualize the affected portion of the brain. **stroke, infarct, contrast material (Haaga, Lee)**

101. **(B)** The canthomeatal line is placed twenty degrees to the scan plane when obtaining pediatric axial sections of the brain. This position avoids the lens of the eye and provides a complete sample of the brain tissue with the least number of scans. **pediatric CT, CT brain (Seeram)**

102. **(D)** The basal ganglia is comprised of gray matter structures that are integrated with the white matter of the cerebrum. The caudate nucleus, claustrum, and the lentiform nucleus which can be subdivided into the putamen and globus pallidus make up the basal ganglia. **cerebrum, basal ganglia (Applegate, Porth)**

103. **(A)** The tentorium cerebelli forms a tent shaped roof over the posterior fossa. The area above the tentorium cerebelli is referred to as the supratentorial region. **tentorium cerebelli, posterior fossa (Applegate, Porth)**

104. **(B)** The third ventricle is illustrated by #3 in Figure 1. **CT brain, ventricles (Applegate, Ellis)**

105. **(D)** The caudate nucleus is illustrated by #1 in Figure 1. **caudate nucleus, basal ganglia (Applegate, Ellis)**

106. **(A)** The anterior horn of the left lateral ventricle is illustrated by #2 in Figure 1. **CT brain, ventricles (Applegate, Ellis)**

107. **(A)** Using a 1mm to 3mm section thickness reduces the possibility of missing a small facial bone fracture. The high resolution algorithm would provide the bony detail to visualize small facial bone fractures. **CT parameters, facial bones, algorithms, kernels (Seeram, Berland, Brooker, Haaga)**

108. **(A)** Because of the combination of high density bone and low density air present in the petrous pyramids a wide window should be selected to cover the large range of CT numbers in this area. The combination of a bone algorithm with small section thickness provide optimal detail for this region. **CT parameters, petrous pyramids, temporal bones (Seeram, Brooker, Haaga)**

109. **(C)** Repositioning of the patient's head and/or changing the gantry angle are acceptable methods of avoiding artifacts from dental fillings. **metallic foreign bodies (Seeram, Haaga)**

110. **(B)** The coronal plane best demonstrates the anatomical relationship between the pituitary gland and the sella turcica. **pituitary gland, sella turcica, coronal imaging (Seeram, Haaga)**

111. **(B)** An epidural hematoma develops between the inner table of the bones of the skull and the dura. It is a direct result of a skull fracture in the temporal bone region of the skull with associated tearing of the middle meningeal artery. **epidural hematoma, fractures of the skull (Porth, Haaga)**

112. **(C)** The Circle of Willis is formed by the internal carotid arteries, anterior cerebral arteries, the anterior communicating artery, the posterior cerebral arteries, and the posterior communicating arteries. **cerebral circulation (Akesson, Applegate)**

113. **(D)** Beam hardening artifacts, metallic objects, and patient motion cause misregistration of the three dimensional reconstructed image. The three dimensional computer program cannot compensate for the depleted image uniformity caused by the above. **artifacts, 3D reconstruction (Seeram, Berland)**

114. **(D)** The amount of contrast material injected, the timing of the CT images with the injection, and the degree of blood brain barrier breakdown influence the intensity of enhancement of an intracranial tumor. **contrast material, intracranial tumors, blood brain barrier (Haaga, Lee)**

115. **(D)** Calcifications have high attenuation values, therefore the calcified pituitary gland has the highest CT number when compared to the other anatomical structures in the ques-

tion. **CT numbers, calcifications (Seeram, Bushong)**

116. **(C)** A beam hardening artifact generally appears as a dark horizontal line between the petrous ridges of the temporal bone. It is commonly referred to as a cupping artifact. **beam hardening artifact, posterior fossa, petrous ridges (Seeram, Haaga)**

117. **(C)** The optic nerve is illustrated by #5 in Figure 2. **optic nerve, coronal imaging (Applegate, Ellis)**

118. **(C)** The maxillary sinus is illustrated be #6 in Figure 2. **maxillary sinus, coronal imaging (Applegate, Ellis)**

119. **(D)** The superior rectus muscle is illustrated by #4 Figure 2. **muscles of the eye, orbit, coronal imaging (Applegate, Ellis)**

120. **(B)** The third ventricle communicates with the fourth ventricle by a long cerebral aqueduct called the aqueduct of sylvius. **ventricles of the brain, cerebral aqueduct (Applegate, Haaga)**

121. **(A)** Axial and direct coronal positioning are routinely performed to obtain axial and coronal images. **patient positioning, direct axial and coronal imaging (Seeram, Haaga)**

122. **(C)** Cerebrospinal fluid is produced in the choroid plexus which originates in the ventricles of the brain. The fluid circulates outward through the fourth ventricle of the brain and into the subarachnoid space around the brain and spinal cord. **cerebrospinal fluid, ventricles of the brain (Applegate, Akesson)**

123. **(A)** Using a thinner section thickness reduces beam hardening artifacts and improves spatial resolution. Radiation dose to the patient is increased. **thin section computed tomography, posterior fossa (Berland, Seeram)**

124. **(D)** Endocrine disease is associated with abnormalities associated with the pituitary gland. Inflammatory disease such as herpes simplex and encephalitis affect the brain. CT of the head is essential in diagnosing hematomas of the brain and imaging fractures involving the

bones of the skull. **CT head, indications (Seeram, Brooker)**

125. **(A)** Subarachnoid hemorrhage most frequently occurs as a result of a ruptured aneurysm. **aneurysms, cerebral hemorrhages (Seeram, Haaga)**

126. **(B)** The orbitomeatal line is placed perpendicular to the tabletop for a lateral scoutview of the head. **routine CT scanning of the head, radiographic positioning baselines (Brooker, Berland)**

127. **(A)** Increasing the gantry angle to compensate for lack of patient neck extension is an acceptable practice. Reformatting axial images is an acceptable option that also decreases the radiation dose to the patient. **CT head, coronal scanning (Brooker, Seeram)**

128. **(D)** Reformatting images reduces the amount of radiation to the patient by eliminating a need for a possible second scanning sequence involving another patient position. It also allows the acquisition of oblique and three dimensional images which is important in evaluating the extent of small facial bone fractures. **multiplanar reformation, maxillofacial trauma (Brooker, Seeram, Haaga)**

129. **(A)** The area that is surveyed on a scoutview of the paranasal sinuses is the base of the skull to the midbrain region. **CT of the paranasal sinuses, scoutview extent (Brooker, Berland)**

130. **(D)** Increasing the mA, kVp, and time will increase contrast resolution, however increasing time can lead to patient motion artifacts. **CT parameters, contrast resolution (Berland, Seeram)**

131. **(C)** Routine scanning of the posterior fossa and the brain begins 1 cm below the base of the skull. **routine positioning, CT of the head, posterior fossa (Berland, Haaga, Brooker)**

132. **(D)** CT scanning of the internal auditory canals includes a scoutview from the base of the skull to the level of the third ventricle. High resolution images are obtained bilaterally for comparison and a 1mm to 2mm section thickness is utilized to maximize spatial resolution. **internal auditory canals , CT parameters (Brooker, Seeram)**

133. **(A)** The zygomatic arch is illustrated by #1 in Figure 3. **zygomatic arch (Ellis, Applegate)**

134. **(B)** The mandibular condyle is illustrated by #3 in Figure 3. **temporomandibular joint, mandibular condyle (Ellis, Applegate)**

135. **(C)** The mastoid air cells are illustrated by #5 in Figure 3. **mastoid air cells, temporal bone (Ellis, Applegate)**

# Neck                                            *(#136-144)*

136. **(C)** Phonation of the letter "E" vibrates the vocal cords, therefore providing definition of vocal cord mobility. **larynx, CT neck procedures (Brooker, Berland)**

137. **(D)** Angling the gantry, extending the chin, and performing both right and left axial obliques are all approved options utilized to avoid artifacts from dental fillings. **CT neck procedures, dental filling artifacts (Brooker, Berland, Seeram)**

138. **(B)** The masseter muscle is illustrated by #1 in Figure 4. **masseter muscle, axial scanning (Ellis, Applegate)**

139. **(B)** The external jugular vein is illustrated by #6 in Figure 4. **vessels of the neck, axial imaging (Ellis, Applegate)**

140. **(D)** The parotid gland is illustrated by #2 in Figure 4. **salivary glands, parotid gland, axial scanning (Ellis, Applegate)**

141. **(B)** Positioning the cervical spine parallel to the axial scanning plane puts the vocal cords in the same plane, therefore the larynx is parallel to the axial plane. **larynx, axial imaging (Berland, Brooker)**

142. **(B)** The lateral is the recommended scout view for routine CT scanning of the neck. **CT neck procedures (Brooker, Berland)**

143. **(A)** The lateral scout view of the neck is taken from T2 to the mid-brain region. **CT neck procedures (Berland, Brooker)**

144. **(C)** The common carotid artery bifurcates into the internal and external carotid arteries at the level of C4-C5. **carotid arteries, bifurcations (Applegate, Akesson)**

# Spine                                            *(#145-177)*

145. **(A)** The examination of one intervertebral disc space should include the region of the pedicle of the vertebra above to the pedicle of the vertebra below. **CT spine, CT procedures (Lee, Brooker)**

146. **(A)** It is recommended that a post myelogram CT be performed 2 to 6 hours after the injection of contrast media. After 6 hrs the concentration of the contrast material dissipates and the contrast media is circulated through the body and eventually excreted. **post myelography CT, contrast media. (Brooker, Haaga, Lee)**

147. **(B)** Intravenous contrast media is not routinely used in spinal CT. It can be used to enhance extramedullary tissues like the dura and blood vessels. Intravenous contrast media can be used to aid in the differentiation of scar tissue from the spinal cord in post laminectomy patients. **CT spine, contrast media (Brooker, Lee)**

148. **(B)** The superior articulating process is illustrated by #3 in Figure 5. **superior articular process, vertebral anatomy (Ellis, Applegate)**

149. **(A)** The transverse process is illustrated by #1 in Figure 5. **transverse process, vertebral anatomy (Ellis, Applegate)**

150. **(B)** The spinous process is illustrated by #5 in Figure 5. **spinous process, vertebral anatomy (Ellis, Applegate)**

151. **(C)** Axial sections are angled to pass parallel through disk spaces since many spinal problems involve the disk or structures that are best assessed in this manner. **spine, procedure (Brooker, Seeram)**

152. **(B)** The spinal cord ends approximately at the L2-L3 vertebral level. The meninges, subarachnoid space, and the cerebrospinal fluid continue to the second sacral segment. **spinal cord (Applegate, Ellis)**

153. **(C)** Contrast media is introduced into the subarachnoid space at a level below the spinal cord. **myelography, post myelography CT of the spine (Ballinger, Lee)**

154. **(C)** 3mm section thickness with 2mm table incrementation provides an overlap of 1mm for each scan. Although, this method improves resolution increases radiation dose to the patient. In newer CT scanners it is possible to reconstruct at overlapping intervals which reduces patient exposure. Overlapping technique provides better information when image reformation into another plane is considered. **cervical spine, procedures (Seeram, Berland)**

155. **(A)** CT is more sensitive and precise than myelography when determining the extent of a lateral disk herniation. L5-S1 disk herniation may not be revealed on myelography. Intrathecal abnormalities such as spinal cord or cauda equinal lesions are best demonstrated by myelography. Cervicothoracic lesions can be obscured due to the position of the shoulders when scanning through this region. It should be stressed that both of these diagnostic tools can easily be used together when diagnosing abnormalities of the spine. **CT of the spine, myelography, procedures (Seeram, Lee, Haaga)**

156. **(C)** The hyoid bone is illustrated by #1 in Figure 6. **hyoid bone, axial imaging (Applegate, Ellis)**

157. **(B)** The lamina of the cervical vertebra is illustrated by #3 in Figure 6. **lamina, cervical anatomy, axial imaging (Haaga, Ellis)**

158. **(B)** The pedicle of the cervical vertebra is illustrated by #5 in Figure 6. **pedicle, cervical anatomy, axial imaging (Ellis, Haaga)**

159. **(B)** The transverse foreman of the cervical vertebra is illustrated by #2 in Figure 6. **transverse foramen, cervical anatomy, axial imaging (Ellis, Applegate)**

160. **(D)** The knees should be flexed as much as possible by placing them over a large foam wedge while removing the arms from the area to be scanned. **procedure, spine (Brooker, Berland)**

161. **(D)** Suspected spinal stenosis, spinal infection, and intraspinal tumors are all indications for spinal computed tomography. **CT spine, indications (Seeram, Lee)**

162. **(D)** Suspended respiration ensures that respiratory motion will not be present and equal inspirations during each scan are usually more comfortable for the patient. **procedure, spine (Brooker, Lee)**

163. **(B)** In cases of disc herniation, there is a focal projection extending from the posterior border. When herniation of a disc occurs it interrupts the symmetrical epidural space the result is a soft tissue density that replaces the lower density of epidural fat. Atrophy of the inferior articular process and lamina is an indicator of spinal stenosis. **herniated nucleus pulposus, CT spine imaging (Haaga, Lee, Porth)**

164. **(B)** The sagittal plane allows the visualization of the relationship between the entire scanned area of the vertebral column and the spinal canal, therefore, the extension of a lesion into the spinal canal can be appreciated to a greater extent. **image reformation, CT of the spine (Lee, Haaga)**

165. **(C)** The lateral scout view allows selection of the scan plane to match the area of interest, usually the disk spaces. **procedure, spine (Brooker, Seeram)**

166. **(D)** By selecting a smaller displayed field of view the operators perception of detail is increased because the size of the image is larger making it easier for the operator to differentiate anatomical references. The displayed image detail is increased, therefore, spatial resolution increases. The anatomy is displayed on a greater number of pixels. The amount of tissue occupied by each pixel is less. **displayed field of view, CT scanning parameters (Berland, Seeram)**

167. **(B)** The ligamentum flavum is illustrated by #3 in Figure 7. **ligamentum flavum, spine (Applegate, Ellis)**

168. **(B)** The apophyseal joint is illustrated by #4 in Figure 7. **apophyseal joint, spine (Applegate, Ellis)**

169. **(B)** The intervertebral disc is illustrated by #1 in Figure 7. **intervertebral disc (Ellis, Applegate)**

170. **(A)** Rolling the patient two or three times before scanning enables the contrast media in the intrathecal space to mix with cerebrospinal fluid therefore, layering of contrast media does not occur and will not cause artifacts on the scan. **contrast media, intrathecal, artifacts (Lee, Haaga)**

171. **(D)** High resolution computed tomography combines thinly collimated sections with a high spatial frequency algorithm that enhances edge detection and with the proper windowing is an excellent tool to evaluate fractures of the spine. Helical/spiral computed tomography scans an entire volume which allows overlapping reconstruction without scanning the patient again. Dynamic scanning is useful in evaluating vascular structures versus intraspinal soft tissue tumors. **acquisition methods, CT spine (Lee, Seeram, Haaga)**

172. **(B)** Helical/Spinal scans an entire volume of tissue. Reconstruction through any arbitrary position within the volume at 0.1mm increments is possible. **acquisition methods, volume scanning (Seeram, Toshiba)**

173. **(B)** Intravenous contrast outlines the epidural venous plexus and intrathecal contrast allows better assessment of the spinal cord and nerve roots. **contrast, protocols (Seeram, Lee)**

174. **(D)** The erector spinae muscle is illustrated by #3 in Figure 8. **erector spinae, spine, muscles (Ellis, Applegate)**

175. **(A)** The costovertebral joint is illustrated by #2 in Figure 8. **costovertebral joint, axial imaging (Ellis, Ballinger)**

176. **(C)** A superficial vascular groove is illustrated by #5 in Figure 8. **vertebral body, vasculature (Lee, Ellis)**

177. **(D)** The crus of the left diaphragm is illustrated by #1 in Figure 8. **spine, axial imaging, crus of the diaphragm (Lee, Ellis)**

# Chest                                                    (#178-222)

178. **(C)** The superior vena cava is illustrated by #2 in figure 9. **superior vena cava, thorax (Ellis, Applegate)**

179. **(A)** The azygos vein is represented by #3 in Figure 9. **azygos vein, thorax (Ellis, Applegate)**

180. **(B)** The descending aorta is illustrated by #4 in Figure 9. **descending aorta, thorax (Ellis, Applegate)**

181. **(A)** Filming of sections is usually done both at window settings for lung and mediastinal structures. **thorax, filming (Berland, Seeram)**

182. **(D)** Contrast enhancement allows visualization of the vasculature of the thorax and its relationship and makes it easy to differentiate an aortic aneurysm from mediastinal masses. Contrast enhancement also helps define the presence and extent of traumatic aneurysms. Contrast enhancement allows visualization of the relationship between a mass and surrounding structures and extension into the mediastinum. **contrast media, CT thorax procedures, aneurysms, mediastinal masses (Seeram, Haaga)**

183. **(A)** Scan extent is defined as the anatomical region that is included during a specific CT examination. When lung carcinoma is suspected it is recommended that the scan begins at the root of the neck which can localized by using the sternal notch as an external landmark and proceeds through the adrenal glands because of the relationship between adrenal carcinomas and lung carcinomas. **CT thorax procedures,scan extent (Berland, Haaga)**

184. **(A)** Visualization of the vasculature of the mediastinum requires an adequate amount of contrast media delivered in a relatively short time frame. A rate of 5 seconds per 50ml is the suggested protocol for imaging the vasculature of the mediastinum when only the bolus technique of injection is performed. The potential of contrast media toxicity must be taken into account. **contrast media, injection rate, mediastinal vasculature (Brooker, Adler)**

185. **(C)** The thorax begins at the root of the neck and extends into the abdomen where the bases of the lungs are found. **thorax, procedure, scout view (Brooker, Berland)**

186. **(C)** The left atrium is illustrated by #4 in Figure 10. **left atrium, heart, axial imaging (Ellis, Applegate)**

187. **(B)** The ascending aorta is illustrated by #3 in Figure 10. **ascending aorta, axial imaging, mediastinal vasculature (Ellis, Applegate)**

188. **(A)** The left ventricle is illustrated by #1 in figure 10. **left ventricle, heart, axial imaging (Ellis, Applegate)**

189. **(C)** A pneumothorax is the most substantial risk involved in a aspiration biopsy of the lung. The patient is monitored by obtaining either a single chest radiograph or a series of chest radiographs if a problem is evident. **aspiration biopsy, pneumothorax (Lee, Haaga)**

190. **(D)** The heart, the great vessels, and the thymus are all parts of the mediastinum. **thorax, mediastinum (Applegate, Lee)**

191. **(A)** The supine position is the most comfortable for the patient and allows for minimal motion of the body from respiration. **thorax, patient positioning (Brooker, Seeram)**

192. **(C)** The pleural cavity is a potential space between the layers of pleura. The right and left pleural cavities are separated and are closed. Air does not move freely in and out during respiration. **pleural cavity, lungs (Applegate, Akesson)**

193. **(C)** The right mainstem bronchus is illustrated by #3 in Figure 11. **main stem bronchi, axial imaging (Ellis, Haaga)**

194. **(B)** The carina is illustrated by #5 in Figure 11. **carina, axial imaging (Ellis, Applegate)**

195. **(A)** The superior vena cava is illustrated by #2 in Figure 11. **superior vena cava, axial imaging (Ellis, Haaga)**

196. **(D)** Lowering the mAs is permissible for CT scanning of the thorax because of the intrinsically high contrast differences of the anatomical tissue differences in the chest. Selecting a half scan mode may permit a longer dynamic scanning sequence. Dynamic scanning sequence is necessary for scanning of the mediastinum and hila and non-dynamic scanning is sufficient for sections below the above regions. **scanning parameters, dynamic scanning, CT chest (Berland, Seeram)**

197. **(C)** Ultrafast (electron beam) CT can produce thirty-four sections per second at 0.1mm increments, therefore it can produce high resolution images of moving organs like the heart. **ultrafast CT, imaging of the heart (Seeram, Berland)**

198. **(C)** A pneumothorax is demonstrated by #1 in figure 12. **pneumothorax, axial imaging (Haaga, Lee)**

199. **(D)** 1600 window width and -600 window level would be the windowing technique that would best correlate with Figure 12. **windowing techniques, lung parenchyma (Seeram, Lee)**

200. **(D)** Increased intercapillary pressure caused by congestive heart causes fluid overload in the capillaries. The fluid permeates or "spills over" into the pleural space. Pleural effusion can also be cause by atelectasis and impaired lymphatic drainage of the pleural space which is usually caused by an obstructive lesion. **pleural effusion, mechanisms of pleural effusions (Porth, Lee)**

201. **(B)** Tissue outside the scanned field of view creates artifacts. The tissue that is not included in the scanned field of view contributes to the image in a negative fashion due to the inaccuracy of CT numbers because of interference with reference detectors. **artifacts, scanned field of view (Berland, Seeram)**

202. **(C)** The arms should not be placed above the patient's head so that they are in the scanned field of view or they will cause artifacts. They must also be placed so as not to interfere with venous drainage. **thorax, chest, contrast, preparation (Brooker, Seeram)**

203. **(D)** Prothrombin time, partial prothrombin time, and platelet count results should be evaluated before any biopsy procedure is performed. **prothrombin time, platelet count, biopsy procedures (Lee, Haaga, Adler)**

204. **(A)** The azygos vein arches over the root of the right lung and enters the superior vena cava. The superior vena cava is formed by the union of the right and left brachiocephalic veins and enters the right atrium. **superior vena cava, vessels of the heart (Applegate, Porth)**

205. **(A)** The right brachiocephalic vein is illustrated by #1 in Figure 13. **mediastinal vasculature, axial imaging (Ellis, Applegate)**

206. **(C)** The trachea is illustrated by #6 in Figure 13. **mediastinum, axial imaging (Ellis, Lee)**

207. **(C)** The left common carotid artery is illustrated by #4 in Figure 13. **mediastinal vasculature, axial imaging (Ellis, Haaga)**

208. **(C)** A narrow window width (400) and a window level of 50 would best demonstrate the structures of the mediastinum. **windowing, mediastinum (Seeram, Berland)**

209. **(D)** A dissecting aortic aneurysm is the result of a break of the tunica intima. The lining coat of an artery is displaced inward creating true and false channels. **dissecting aortic aneurysm, procedures (Webb, Lee)**

210. **(D)** Computed tomography of the thorax is indicated for the detection of pulmonary masses, to define pleural tumor extent, and to determine if a pulmonary infiltrate is an abscess or resolving pneumonia. **indications, CT thorax, procedures (Lee, Haaga)**

211. **(D)** Thicker sections are adequate for survey studies and decrease the overall number of sections needed to cover the chest. **thorax, procedure, section factors (Berland, Brooker, Seeram)**

212. **(D)** The right pulmonary artery is illustrated by #3 in Figure 14. **pulmonary vessels, axial imaging (Ellis, Lee)**

213. **(D)** The pulmonary trunk is illustrated by #1 in Figure 14. **pulmonary vessels, axial imaging (Ellis, Applegate)**

214. **(C)** The superior vena cava is illustrated by #4 in Figure 14. **superior vena cava, axial imaging (Ellis, Lee)**

215. **(D)** Standard inspirations are more equal and standard in volume and inspirations of this type demonstrate the lung and mediastinum without increasing their overall length. **procedure, chest, thorax (Berland, Seeram, Lee)**

216. **(B)** High resolution computed tomography to examine the lung parenchyma should include thinly collimated sections (1-2mm), a high frequency spatial algorithm that enhances edge detection, and a reduced displayed field of view to cover the lung parenchyma only, maximizing detail. **high resolution computed tomography, lung parenchyma, procedures (Seeram, Haaga, Berland)**

217. **(D)** The preferred injection site to introduce contrast media for CT examination of the chest is in the left arm at a medially situated antecubital vein. This technique optimizes opacification of the left brachiocephalic vein and provides a direct route to the right brachiocephalic vein which empties directly into the superior vena cava. Antecubital refers to the elbow region. **antecubital veins, contrast media routes, procedures (Seeram, Adler)**

218. **(D)** Helical/spiral CT is superior to dynamic (rapid) sequential scanning. Helical/spiral CT scans entire volumes of tissue in a single breath, thereby eliminating any interscan or intergroup delay necessary for table indexing and mechanical delays for dynamic scanning. Motion artifacts due to inconsistent levels of respiration which leads to image misregistration of multiplanar reconstruction and 3D processing are eliminated. **helical/spiral CT, volume scanning (Seeram, Toshiba)**

219. **(C)** A pathological process is illustrated by #2 in Figure 15. **mediastinum, thorax, pathology (Lee, Haaga)**

220. **(B)** A pathological process is illustrated by #4 in Figure 15. **mediastinum, thorax, pathology (Lee, Haaga)**

221. **(B)** The descending aorta is illustrated by #1 in Figure 15. **mediastinal vessels, axial imaging (Ellis, Lee)**

222. **(D)** The pectoralis major is an anterior superficial muscle of the thorax. The trapezius is a posterior superficial muscle of the thorax. The latissimus dorsi is a lateral superficial muscle of the thorax. **thorax musculature (Applegate, Akesson)**

# Abdomen                                         *(#223-267)*

223. **(A)** Oral contrast given 1 to 2 hours before the exam will fill the entire small bowel of most patients and a second dose given just prior to the exam will fill the proximal

bowel and stomach. **contrast, procedure, abdomen (Berland, Brooker, Seeram)**

224. **(A)** The percentage of barium in a barium sulfate suspension is 1-3% for abdominal computed tomography. **barium sulfate suspension, abdominal CT (Seeram, Lee, Haaga)**

225. **(A)** Oral water soluble contrast media is indicated when the use of barium is contraindicated and it is utilized by many radiology departments are part of the routine. Water soluble and barium sulfate result in comparable bowel opacification. **water soluble contrast media, abdominal CT (Lee, Berland)**

226. **(D)** Oral contrast media distends the intestinal lumen that is necessary to estimate wall thickness. Nonspecific, mural thickening is an important indicator of a gastrointestinal abnormality. Oral contrast helps distinguish loops of bowel from abnormal abdominal fluid collection and masses. **oral contrast media, indications, abdominal CT (Lee, Haaga, Seeram)**

227. **(A)** The ligamentum teres is illustrated by #1 in Figure 16. **hepatic ligaments, axial imaging of the liver (Ellis, Applegate)**

228. **(B)** The left adrenal gland is illustrated by #3 in Figure 16. **suprarenal gland, axial imaging (Ellis, Applegate)**

229. **(B)** The superior mesenteric artery is illustrated by #2 in Figure 16. **superior mesenteric artery, visceral branches of the abdominal aorta (Ellis, Applegate)**

230. **(B)** The structures to be included for a routine abdomen exam all lie between the base of the lungs and the iliac crests. **abdomen, scout view (Seeram, Haaga)**

231. **(D)** The pancreas, duodenum, and the kidneys are retroperitoneal structures. These structures are located behind the peritoneum. **retroperitoneal anatomy, peritoneum (Applegate, Haaga)**

232. **(C)** Percutaneous needle biopsy is indicated for determining the nature of an abnormality, staging of intraabdominal malignancies. Localization of a specific lesion

should be done prior to a needle biopsy. **needle biopsy, procedures (Lee, Haaga)**

233. **(B)** When contrast media reaches the tubules of the kidney opacification of the medullary region occurs. The normal time frame is 1 to 3 minutes. It is at this time that maximum opacification of the kidney occurs. **kidney, intravenous contrast media, procedures (Lee, Haaga)**

234. **(A)** 1ml/kg is an acceptable dose of intravenous contrast media for a pediatric CT of the abdomen. Additional contrast media administration depends on the specific area being evaluated, weight, and age of the patient. **contrast media, pediatric procedures (Haaga, Lee, Seeram)**

235. **(D)** The length of the normal adrenal gland is variable but is usually 2 to 6cm in length and 5 to 6mm thick. The adrenal gland is relatively small, therefore, patient respiration, bowel peristalsis and surgical clips can cause artifacts on the scan making it difficult to evaluate the adrenal glans. **image misregistration, artifacts, adrenal glands (Haaga, Berland, Lee)**

236. **(D)** The pharmacokinetics which occur following a sustained bolus injection are described by three distinct phases, the bolus phase, the nonequilibrium phase, and the equilibrium phase. The phases are of importance for the CT evaluation of the liver. Pharmacokinetics is the study of the metabolism and action of drugs, contrast media, with emphasis on absorption time, duration of action, distribution in the body, and method of excretion. **pharmacokinetics, contrast media, CT liver procedures (Lee, Haaga)**

237. **(B)** The splenic flexure of the colon is illustrated by #4 in Figure 17. **colon, large intestine, axial imaging (Ellis, Applegate)**

238. **(A)** The gallbladder is illustrated by #1 in Figure 17. **gallbladder, axial imaging (Ellis, Applegate)**

239. **(C)** The fundus portion of the stomach is illustrated by #6 in Figure 17. **stomach, axial imaging (Ellis, Applegate)**

240. **(D)** Rescanning the patient 4 to 6 hrs after a full injection of contrast media aids in the visualization of liver lesions. The liver remains enhanced due to hepatic excretion while lesions return to normal density. Refilming the case using a narrower window width will reduce the range of gray scale but is useful to display subtle density differences in the liver. The bolus injection technique with rapid scanning aids in the determination of vascular involvement and lesion boarders within the liver. **liver, procedures (Seeram, Haaga, Lee)**

241. **(B)** Relaxed suspended expiration is recommended for routine abdominal scanning. **procedures (Berland, Lee)**

242. **(B)** The common bile duct is formed by the union of the common hepatic duct and cystic duct. **digestive system, gallbladder, liver (Ballinger, Applegate)**

243. **(A)** It is recommended that 5mm section thickness be combined with a 5mm couch index for routine scanning of the pancreas. If a lesion is localized smaller section thickness and table index is recommended. **pancreas, procedures (Seeram, Lee)**

244. **(C)** The portal vein is illustrated by #3 in Figure 18. **portal vein, axial imaging (Lee, Haaga)**

245. **(B)** The tail of the pancreas is illustrated by #5 in Figure 18. **pancreas, axial imaging (Haaga, Lee)**

246. **(B)** The spleen is illustrated by #1 in Figure 18. **spleen, axial imaging (Lee, Haaga)**

247. **(C)** The right lateral decubitus position will aid in the filling of the duodenum, Therefore the head of the pancreas can be distinguished from the duodenum. **pancreas, procedures (Brooker, Haaga)**

248. **(A)** CT is the method of choice when evaluating the retroperitoneum because the area scanned is not obscured by bowel gas or fat especially in the axial plane. **retroperitoneum, ultrasound, CT procedures (Seeram, Lee, Webb)**

249. **(C)** A selection of a low frequency spatial algorithm can be used for smoothing, which can improve lesion perceptibility. Collimation determines section thickness.

Thinner section thickness utilizes narrow collimation, which reduces scatter intercepted by the detectors. Decreasing the mAs, decreases photon flux which adversely effects contrast resolution. **contrast resolution, procedures (Seeram, Berland)**

250. **(A)** Hemangiomas and adenomas are benign lesions. adenocarcinomas are malignant. **pathology, liver (Porth, Haaga)**

251. **(C)** CT arteriography and CT arterial portography are two techniques that have improved the detection of liver lesions. Contrast media can be introduced via a catheter in either the hepatic or superior mesenteric artery. **CT arteriography, celiac axis, procedures (Seeram, Haaga)**

252. **(A)** The left renal artery is illustrated by #1 in Figure 19. **renal arteries, axial imaging (Ellis, Lee)**

253. **(B)** The left renal vein is illustrated by #4 in Figure 19. **renal veins, axial imaging (Ellis, Haaga)**

254. **(D)** The abdominal aorta is illustrated by #2 in Figure 19. **abdominal aorta, axial imaging (Ellis, Applegate)**

255. **(D)** Keeping the patient NPO after midnight the night before abdominal scanning allows ample time for the digestive tract to digest foods therefore, minimizing the chance of vomiting and aspiration when intravenous contrast media is administered. Ingestion of the oral contrast material is ingested more easily because the stomach is not full and it minimizes the chance of diagnostic confusion between masses and undigested food particles. **oral contrast administration, procedures (Berland, Brooker)**

256. **(A)** The greatest value of a pre-intravenous contrast abdominal scan is to determine specific levels for an intravenous contrast dynamic scan technique. **pre-intravenous contrast scan, dynamic scanning, procedures (Haaga, Lee)**

257. **(C)** Helical/spiral computed tomography would provide the best results for trauma abdominal scanning. Helical/spiral CT provides a greater area to be scanned in the shortest amount of time. There is superior cover-

age of the z-axis which is the direction of the table movement. By extending the helix, resolution is not compromised due to the interpolation method of reconstruction. Helical/spiral CT can reconstruct an image at any arbitrary location at 0.1mm incrementation. Continuous scanning in a single breath is possible and interscan delays are eliminated. **helical/spiral CT, procedures (Seeram, Toshiba)**

258. **(D)** Malignant neoplasms metastasize by seeding within the body cavities, lymphatic spread, and embolistic spread. **metastasis (Porth, Lee)**

259. **(D)** The spleen is a retroperitoneal structure and is located posteriorly in the abdomen. When coronal images are obtained the spleen would be visualized first if the images were reformatted from posterior to anterior. **coronal imaging, spleen (Applegate, Ellis, Lee)**

260. **(A)** The head of the pancreas is the most anteriorly positioned of the anatomical structures listed in question 260. **head of the pancreas, anatomical position (Ellis, Applegate)**

261. **(C)** When obtaining sagittal images from right to left the gallbladder would be visualized first of the anatomical structures listed in question 261. **gallbladder, sagittal imaging (Ellis, Applegate)**

262. **(A)** The splenic and superior mesenteric veins join to form the portal vein. **portal circulation (Haaga, Applegate)**

263. **(D)** Fractures of the kidney, subcapsular hematomas, and retroperitoneal hemorrhages can be demonstrated by abdominal computed tomography. **abdominal trauma, procedures (Lee, Haaga)**

264. **(D)** Streak artifacts caused be ribs, lack of homogeneous contrast enhancement of the spleen, streak artifacts caused by oral contrast media can obscure portions of the spleen during CT scanning. **CT of the spleen, artifacts (Haaga, Lee)**

265. **(D)** The air filled fundus of the stomach is illustrated by #1 in Figure 20. **fundus of the stomach, axial imaging (Ellis, Lee)**

266. **(A)** An attenuation value of 3.5 represents a fluid consistency. The location is in the location around the liver, therefore ascites is most likely represented. **ascites, liver (Haaga, Lee)**

267. **(B)** The spleen is illustrated by #3 in Figure 20. **spleen, axial imaging (Haaga, Ellis)**

# Pelvis *(#268-303)*

268. **(A)** The scan extent for a routine examination of the pelvis would commence from the iliac crest and conclude at the symphysis pubis. **CT pelvis, procedures (Lee, Berland)**

269. **(C)** The uterus is an oval structure that is viewed in the axial plane slightly indenting the posterior aspect of the bladder. The vaginal orifice, rectum, and the sacrum are all positioned posteriorly to the uterus respectively. **uterus, axial imaging, pelvic structures (Applegate, Ellis)**

270. **(A)** Without the use of a tampon the vagina is collapsed and appears as soft tissue mass between the bladder and the rectum. Insertion of a tampon distends the vaginal canal and helps to locate the cervix and uterus. **CT of the female pelvis, procedures (Haaga, Lee, Seeram)**

271. **(A)** Visualization of the distal colon can be accomplished by giving 500cc's of oral contrast the night before the exam. The distal colon may also be visualized via a contrast enema of 300-500cc's. Giving 300-500cc's of oral contrast 30 minutes prior to the exam would provide an inadequate amount of time for the contrast to reach the distal colon. **CT of the pelvis, contrast media, procedures (Berland, Brooker)**

272. **(C)** Direct coronal imaging of the floor of the pelvis is the best method of evaluation. **CT of the pelvis, coronal imaging, procedures (Haaga, Lee)**

273. **(B)** The epididymis and the testes are located within the male scrotum. The seminal vesicles are located posterior to the bladder and superior to the prostate. **reproductive system, male pelvis (Haaga, Applegate)**

274. **(B)** The abdominal aorta bifurcates into the right and left common iliac arteries at the L4 vertebral level. The

common iliac arteries then divide into the internal and external iliac arteries. **pelvic vasculature, arteries (Applegate, Akesson)**

275. **(B)** The external iliac vein is illustrated by #6 in Figure 21. **CT pelvis, vasculature, axial imaging (Applegate, Ellis)**

276. **(D)** The contrast enhanced left ureter is illustrated by #3 in Figure 21. **CT pelvis, ureters, axial imaging (Ellis, Haaga)**

277. **(A)** The urinary bladder is illustrated by #1 in Figure 21. **CT pelvis, urinary bladder, axial imaging (Ellis, Applegate)**

278. **(D)** Visualization of the urinary bladder can be accomplished with the introduction of either positive or negative contrast media. Iodinated contrast media can be given either intravenously or via a foley catheter. Carbon dioxide can be introduced via a foley catheter and is utilized to visualize small lesions of the wall of the bladder. Carbon dioxide is more readily absorbed by the body than room air. **contrast media, urinary bladder, procedures (Haaga, Lee, Seeram)**

279. **(B)** Computed tomography can readily determine the extent of a known malignancy and the surrounding structures and involvement of pelvic lymph nodes. CT also is chosen instead of ultrasound when a pelvic abscess contains gas because of the echogenic problems associated with a sound beam and gas. **CT of the female pelvis, procedures (Haaga, Lee)**

280. **(A)** Urine acts as a natural contrast for the bladder during pelvis exams. **bladder, preparation (Berland, Seeram)**

281. **(A)** The seminal vesicle is illustrated by #1 in Figure 22. **CT male pelvis, seminal vesicle, axial imaging (Haaga, Ellis)**

282. **(C)** The gluteus maximus muscle is illustrated by #2 in Figure 22. **pelvic musculature, axial imaging (Ellis, Applegate)**

283. **(B)** The rectum is illustrated by #3 in Figure 22. **rectum, axial imaging (Ellis, Lee)**

284. **(A)** The terms used to describe the region below the pelvic brim are the true pelvis which also is known as the lesser pelvis. **true pelvis, anatomical divisions (Haaga, Applegate, Akesson)**

285. **(B)** A ventral hernia occurs when fat and bowel protrude anteriorly through the linea alba. **pelvic herniations, linea alba (Haaga, Lee, Porth)**

286. **(D)** The ascending colon would be visualized first of the structure listed in question 286 when obtaining sagittal sections from right to left. **large intestine, sagittal reformation (Applegate, Akesson)**

287. **(A)** The primary clinical role of computed tomography for carcinoma of the bladder is to determine the presence of invasion of perivesicle fat, adjacent viscera, and pelvic lymph nodes. CT cannot determine microscopic invasion, and superficial lesions from one another. An intravenous urogram or a cystogram would be the screening procedure of choice. **CT of the pelvis, urinary bladder, pathology (Haaga, Lee, Wolbarst)**

288. **(A)** Iodinated contrast media concentrations of 20 - 30% would provide acceptable visualization of the urinary bladder. The higher the percentage the denser the urinary bladder becomes, therefore, the greater the chance of scan artifacts occurring. **contrast media, CT of the urinary bladder, procedures (Haaga, Lee, Adler)**

289. **(D)** Localization of lesions for radiation therapy planning, determining the stage of prostate neoplasms, and evaluating response to chemotherapy are all clinical indications for the use of computed tomography of the pelvis. **CT of the pelvis, indications, procedures (Haaga, Lee, Wolbarst)**

290. **(B)** The prostate gland is illustrated by #4 in Figure 23. **prostate gland, axial imaging (Ellis, Applegate)**

291. **(B)** The ischium is illustrated by #3 in Figure 23. **ischium, bony pelvis, axial imaging (Ellis, Applegate)**

292. **(C)** The rectum is illustrated by #2 in Figure 23. **rectum, axial imaging (Ellis, Applegate)**

293  (A)  An AP scoutview is recommended for a routine examination of the pelvis. **CT of the pelvis, procedures (Lee, Berland)**

294.  (C)  An edge gradient artifact is a streak artifact caused by tangentially oriented object like a biopsy needle or an obliquely oriented anatomical structure such as the pelvic bone. **artifacts, edge gradient (Berland, Seeram)**

295.  (C)  The rectouterine pouch is located between the uterus and rectum and is also known as Douglas's pouch. **female pelvic anatomy (Akesson, Applegate)**

296.  (B)  The problem is solved in two steps. First, solve for pitch. Pitch equals couch top speed divided by section thickness. 10mm/sec divided by 10mm equals a pitch of 1. Secondly, solve for the total volume scanned. Total volume scanned is equal to pitch X section thickness X rotations per second X total scan time. 1 x 10 x 1/sec x 20 seconds equals 200mm total volume scanned. **helical/spiral, volume scanning, pitch, total volume (Toshiba, Seeram)**

297.  (D)  The undescended testicle is generally visualized as an oval or round soft tissue density that can be as small 1cm. unopacified bowel loops, vascular structures, and lymph nodes can make the visualization of an undescended testicle difficult in the upper pelvis. **CT of the pelvis, undescended testicle (Haaga, Lee)**

298.  (A)  When invasion of bony structures from a soft tissue mass is suspected it is essential that the study be filmed using two window widths and window levels. 350/WW, 350/WL would adequately image the soft tissue. 2000/WW, 200/WL would adequately image the bony structures. **windowing, soft tissue, bone Seeram, Haaga, Lee)**

299.  (C)  When too low of an mAs value is selected for the pelvis low contrast detectability decreases which results in loss of detail. **contrast resolution, low contrast detectability, scanning parameters (Berland, Seeram)**

300.  (A)  If a patient is not centered properly detectors may be blocked causing out of field artifacts and inaccurate CT numbers. **CT numbers, artifacts, patient positioning (Berland, Seeram)**

301. **(B)** A CT number of 0 equals a water density. A cyst typically is a round well defined structure and if it has an attenuation of 0 it is a cyst. A uterine cyst is illustrated by #1 in Figure 23. **cysts, CT numbers (Haaga, Lee, Wolbarst)**

302. **(B)** The right sacroiliac joint is illustrated by #3 in Figure 23. **sacroiliac joint, axial imaging (Applegate, Ellis)**

303. **(A)** The uterus is illustrated by #2 in Figure 23. **uterus axial imaging (Ellis, Applegate)**

# Musculoskeletal                                    (#304-315)

304. **(A)** The AP pelvic scout view is recommended for CT of the acetabular region. **scout view, acetabulum (Berland, Haaga, Lee)**

305. **(D)** Minimal positioning maneuvers, defining the extent of complicated fractures, and manipulation of acquired data such as windowing techniques and multiplanar reformation makes CT the desired modality for imaging of trauma to the musculoskeletal system. **trauma CT, musculoskeletal system (Haaga, Lee, Seeram)**

306. **(B)** The patient is placed in a supine position with the hands supinated. This action places the shoulders and scapulae in anatomical position. **CT of the shoulders and scapulae, positioning (Haaga, Lee)**

307. **(C)** The intercondyloid fossa is illustrated by #4 in Figure 25. **knee, axial imaging (Ellis, Applegate)**

308. **(C)** The medial head of the gastrocnemius muscle is illustrated by #3 in Figure 25. **knee, musculature, axial imaging (Ellis, Applegate)**

309. **(A)** The lateral condyle of the right femur is illustrated by #5 in Figure 25. **femur, axial imaging (Ellis, Applegate)**

310. **(B)** Elimination of patient motion and thin overlapping sections of the are of interest are a requirement for 3D reconstruction. **3D reconstruction, procedures (Seeram, Berland)**

311. **(C)** When a mass is located on an initial screening exam a second scan should be performed utilizing thin sections. Both upper extremities should be symmetrically positioned for accurate comparison. An injection of contrast media below the mass allows for complete circulation which enables enhancement of all of the surrounding vasculature. **CT of the upper extremity, procedures (Haaga, Lee)**

312. **(D)** Computed tomography is superior to angiography when evaluating soft tissues and lesions and it's relationship to surrounding vasculature. Nuclear medicine bone scans do not provide complete and exact determination of soft tissue position relative to bone. Computed tomography can image complicated intraarticular fractures that may be superimposed on conventional radiography. **modalities, procedures (Haaga, Lee, Seeram)**

313. **(A)** The acromion process is illustrated by #4 in Figure 26. **CT of the shoulder and scapula, axial imaging (Applegate, Akesson)**

314. **(C)** The glenoid is illustrated by #1 in Figure 26. **CT of the shoulder and scapula, axial imaging (Applegate, Akesson)**

315. **(D)** A fractured clavicle is illustrated by #5 in Figure 26. **clavicle, axial imaging (Applegate, Ellis)**

# Physics and
# Instrumentation    *(#316 - 450)*

## System Operation & Components    *(#316 - 342)*

316.  **(D)**   Xenon gas under pressure is most commonly used in gas-filled ionization chamber detectors. **computed tomography detectors, ionization chambers (Berland, Seeram, Brooker, Carlton, Bushberg, Wolbarst, Bushong, Curry)**

317.  **(D)**   The efficiency range of solid state crystal detectors is 95 - 99%. **computed tomography detectors, ionization chambers (Berland, Carlton)**

318.  **(B)**   The translation motion was eliminated in the third generation scanners. Detector signal drift sensitivity and spurious signals from moving signal wires were problems that were acquired by third generation scanners. Third generation scanners were also more expensive. **computed tomography generation configurations, detectors (Berland, Carlton, Bushberg)**

319.  **(A)**   X-ray tube output level and anode heat load design are fundamental considerations for tube life. Greater loads (mA level, time of exposures, number of exposure) will decrease tube life. The greater the number of heat units the tube anode can handle, the greater the tube life. Cathode to anode distance is not a significant factor. **x-ray tubes, computed tomography tubes, x-ray source (Berland, Carlton, Bushong)**

320.  **(A)**   Information is lost when an analog signal is digitized. However, the digital signal can later be returned to an analog state (although with reduced information) and the resulting information can be handled by a computer processing system. In fact, computers require digital information for processing applications. **digital**

processing, computer processing (Carlton, Berland, Bushberg, Seeram)

321. **(D)** Optical disk, optical tape, and magnetic tape, as well as magnetic disks, are all capable of storing computed tomography data. **digital processing, computer processing, data storage (Carlton, Seeram, Bushong)**

322. **(D)** All three descriptions are true regarding solid state scintillation detectors. They have better absorption efficiency than xenon detectors (it is near 100%). They are the only type of detector that can be used in a fourth generation system with changing tube to detector alignment because they can accept photons from varying angles. They have poor scatter rejection ability, also because they accept photons from varying angles. **detectors, scintillation detectors, solid state detectors (Bushberg, Seeram, Berland)**

323. **(D)** The table, patient, and x-ray tube are all in motion during an exposure with a helical or spiral computed tomography unit. **computed tomography: helix, helical, spiral (Bushberg, Seeram, Toshiba)**

324. **(D)** Pitch is defined as: the table increment in distance per mm per 360° gantry rotation divided by the section thickness in mm for a helical or spiral scanner. **computed tomography: helix, helical, spiral (Bushberg, Seeram)**

325. **(A)** Nutation (a nutating motion) comes from astronomy where it is used to describe orbital wobble. In computed tomography the term describes a tube and detector configuration where the tube rotates 360° while a 360° ring of detectors angles out of path of the x-ray tube. **nutation, computed tomography generation configurations, detectors (Berland, Carlton, Bushberg)**

326. **(D)** The kVp level, tissue density and tissue thickness will all increase the x-ray beam hardening. Beam hardening is defined as increasing the average keV of photons reaching the detectors. Increased kVp will increase the quantity of higher keV photons. Both tissue density and thickness accomplish this by absorbing lower keV photons. **x-ray source, exposure, filtration (Berland, Carlton, Bushong, Wolbarst)**

327. **(B)** Array processors increase display speed by decreasing processing time. They do not increase the data available for window width processing. That is a function of the quantity of data received by the detector. **array processors, digital processing, computer processing (Carlton, Berland, Bushberg, Seeram)**

328. **(A)** Sodium iodide and cesium iodide have been replaced by bismuth germanate, calcium fluoride, and gadolinium based ceramic materials in scintillation CT detectors. **computed tomography detectors, ionization chambers (Wolbarst, Seeram, Carlton, Bushberg)**

329. **(D)** Air gap, fixed grids, and source collimation have all been used to reduce the scatter radiation received by the detectors. **collimation, scatter, detectors (Berland, Bushberg)**

330. **(C)** The bus is a conduit for the transfer of information from one component to another. **computer, central processing unit, digital processing (Carlton, Wolbarst, Bushong, Seeram)**

331. **(C)** Incident beam collimation determines section thickness. **collimation, section thickness (Berland, Carlton, Bushberg, Bushong, Wolbarst)**

332. **(D)** Patient exposure does not limit dynamic scanning time. However, the interscan delay, scan duration, and tube heat loading capacity do limit dynamic scanning time. **dynamic scanning (Berland, Bushberg, Seeram)**

333. **(C)** (P) Pitch = (I) table increment in mm per 360° gantry rotation ÷ (S) section thickness in mm. $P = I/S$ or $S = I/P$ or $S = 15$ mm/1.2 or $S = 12.5$ mm. **computed tomography: helix, helical, spiral (Bushberg, Seeram, Picker, Toshiba)**

334. **(A)** Read only memory (ROM) is computer memory that cannot be used for data storage because it contains basic operating instructions for the system. RAM is random access memory, which is used to store data. A CPU is the central processing unit while a CRT is a cathode ray tube or viewing monitor. **computer, computer memory, read only memory (Carlton, Seeram, Bushong, Wolbarst)**

335. **(C)** Both radiation exposure to the patient and x-ray tube heating are proportional to mAs because mAs controls the quantity of photons exiting the tube. The length of scan time is inversely proportional to mAs. **x-ray tubes, x-ray source, exposure to patient, milliampere-seconds (Berland, Carlton, Bushong, Bushberg, Wolbarst)**

336. **(B)** Once secondary scatter has been produced, it is prevented from reaching the detectors by post-patient collimation. Pre-patient collimation, fine slit collimation, and beam shaping filters are used to reduce the amount of primary beam reaching the patient, which reduces the amount of secondary scatter produced in the first place. **collimation, scatter radiation (Bushberg, Berland, Seeram)**

337. **(A)** A pitch of 0.8 would produce oversampling of data with a helical or spiral scanner. A pitch of 1.0 provides table movement equal to the section thickness. A pitch of less than 1.0 oversamples a portion of each section. **computed tomography: helix, helical, spiral (Bushberg, Seeram, Picker, Toshiba)**

338. **(B)** A track ball and keyboard are input devices to the central processing unit (CPU). A laser film printer is an output device. **computer, input devices, peripherals (Carlton, Seeram, Bushong)**

339. **(D)** Shorter scan times, single breath hold technique for many procedures eliminating variation from differences in breath holding, and the need for less contrast media are all advantages of helical or spiral computed tomography units. **computed tomography: helix, helical, spiral (Bushberg, Seeram)**

340. **(C)** Xenon gas under a pressure of 20 - 25 atmospheres (atm) is most commonly used in gas-filled ionization chamber detectors. **computed tomography detectors, ionization chambers (Berland, Seeram, Brooker, Carlton, Bushberg, Wolbarst, Bushong, Curry)**

341. **(D)** The scanning speed, quality of amplifiers, and the speed of the computer acquisition system all are effected by a decision to use a pulsed or continuous output x-ray tube. Although a pulsed system will conserve the life of the x-ray tube, scanning speed will be reduced. Increased amplifier quality will permit the

use of a pulsed system, as will a faster computer (data) acquisition system. **x-ray source (Berland, Seeram)**

342. **(A)** An array processor failure would increase image display time because the other processors and/or main computer would have to assume the functions normally done by the failed processor. **digital processing, computer processing, array processor (Seeram, Carlton, Bushong, Bushberg)**

## Image Processing & Display *(#343-390)*

343. **(C)** A pixel is a picture element. **pixel (Seeram, Bushberg, Berland, Wolbarst, Bushong, Carlton, Curry, Hendee)**

344. **(D)** The number of detected photons will double (increase 100%) if a section thickness is changed from 5 mm to 10 mm. **section thickness, collimation (Berland, Bushberg, Seeram)**

345. **(A)** The pencil thin x-ray beam that strikes a single detector is referred to as a ray. The projection or view is the set of rays striking a detector array. **ray, projection, view (Bushberg, Berland, Wolbarst, Seeram)**

346. **(A)** The loss of image that occurs at the edge where each section abuts the next is caused by the relatively large focal spot of the x-ray tube, the edge effect of the collimator (divergence of the beam), and by the x-ray scatter produced in the patient. The reconstruction algorithm does not produce the angled edge described in this question. **acquisition, section thickness, reconstruction (Bushberg, Wolbarst, Seeram)**

347. **(C)** Three-dimensional surface rendering is accomplished by the computer drawing a contour line where the bone to soft tissue interface occurs and then stacking or tiling the contours to give the impression of overlap and depth. **three-dimensional display, three-dimensional rendering (Wolbarst, Seeram, Carlton, Bushberg)**

348. **(B)** Decreasing the field of view will permit true magnification of the image because each pixel represents less tissue. Normal size display therefore magnifies the tissue represented by each pixel. **magnification, field of view (Carlton, Bushberg, Webb, Seeram, Bushnong)**

349. **(C)** There are two broad categories of algorithms, iterative and analytical. The two analytical methods commonly used in computed tomography reconstructions are Fourier and back-projection. **algorithms, back-projection, Fourier (Wolbarst, Seeram, Bushberg, Carlton)**

350. **(D)** The typical range for the maximum angle of rotation for a conventional CT scanner is 450-500°. **image acquisition, number of projections (Bushberg, Wolbarst, Seeram, Carlton)**

351. **(B)** The pixel size is calculated by dividing the field of view by the matrix size. So, 45 cm/512 = 0.09 cm or 0.9 mm. **matrix, field of view, pixel (Berland, Bushberg, Seeram, Carlton, Hendee)**

352. **(D** Air has a negative CT or Hounsfield number. Water is 0. Bone and blood have positive numbers. **CT numbers, Hounsfield numbers (Seeram, Bushberg, Berland, Wolbarst, Bushong, Carlton, Curry, Hendee)**

353. **(A)** When too large a displayed field of view is selected, the size of the anatomical region being examined within the image is reduced. The viewer's perceptibility is decreased. The anatomical region being examined is displayed on fewer pixels therefore, the amount of tissue occupied by each pixel is greater. **displayed field of view, displayed detail, perceptibility (Berland, Seeram)**

354. **(B)** A kernel is the same as a reconstruction filter. **kernel, reconstruction filters (Seeram, Berland)**

355. **(A)** Filtered back-projection is convolution. **convolution, back-projection, analytical reconstruction (Wolbarst, Bushberg, Carlton, Seeram, Bushong)**

356. **(C)** Commonly used matrix sizes include 256 x 256, 320 x 320, 360 x 360, and 512 x 512. There is no 440 x 440 matrix used in computed tomography. **matrix (Berland, Carlton, Hendee, Bushong, Bushberg, Wolbarst, Curry, Seeram)**

357. **(B).** The window width is the range of CT numbers within which the entire gray scale is displayed. The window width determines the maximum number of shades of

gray that can be displayed on a monitor. **window width (Berland, Seeram, Wolbarst, Carlton)**

358. **(C)** There are 262,144 pixels in a 512 X 512 matrix. The answer is derived by multiplying the first number in the size of the matrix by the second number. **matrix, pixel (Seeram, Carlton, Bushberg)**

359. **(A)** The benefits of narrower section thicknesses are reduced partial volume averaging and improved spatial resolution, both due to the decreased volume of tissue in the voxel. Narrower section thicknesses increase scan time. **section thickness, spatial resolution, spatial volume averaging (Berland, Bushberg, Seeram, Carlton, Bushong, Hendee)**

360. **(A)** Stacked contiguous transverse axial images would produce the best results when compared to the other distractors. Non-contiguous or gapped sections could result in a step-like formations which could resemble fractures. **multiplanar reformation, (Seeram, Berland)**

361. **(D)** The linear attenuation coefficient of a material is determined by the density of the material being scanned, the atomic number of the material, the energy of the incident photons penetrating the material. **linear attenuation coefficient (Berland, Seeram, Carlton, Wolbarst)**

362. **(C)** The z-axis of an imaging plane is the longitudinal direction. **z-axis, imaging plane, coordinates (Seeram, Wolbarst, Bushberg)**

363. **(D)** The type of reconstruction algorithm, The size of the matrix, and the rate of analog to digital conversion of detected x-ray signals all have an influence on reconstruction speed. **reconstruction speed (Seeram, Berland)**

364. **(C)** The section sensitivity profile is the descriptor that is used to graphically quantify section thickness. In conventional CT the perfect section sensitivity profile would be that a 10mm section thickness actually equals 10mm. Because of geometric unsharpness and scatter the perfect scenario does not occur. **section sensitivity profile, section thickness (Haaga, Picker, Bushberg)**

365. **(A)** The approximate resolving ability of most cathode ray tube (CRT) viewing monitors is in the range of 1-2 lp/mm. **digital image acquisition, cathode ray tubes, monitors (Carlton, Curry, Seeram)**

366. **(B)** Water is represented by a CT or Hounsfield number of 0. **CT numbers, Hounsfield numbers (Seeram, Bushberg, Berland, Wolbarst, Bushong, Carlton, Curry, Hendee)**

367. **(B)** Partial volume averaging is when two or more attenuation values are contained within one voxel. The voxel would have a CT number that is based on an average of the attenuation values of the CT numbers that are represented. **partial volume averaging (Berland, Seeram, Wolbarst, Bushberg)**

368. **(A)** There are a number of quality assurance tests for determining resolution performance of a CT scanner. Some of the factors that could cause a scanner to fail one of these tests are detector vibrations, decreased tube output, and increased electronic noise. **resolution, QA testing (Seeram, Bushberg, Carlton, Berland)**

369. **(B)** Milliamperage should be increased or decrease depending what type of change is done to section thickness and scanning speed if radiation dose is not a factor. **milliamperage, section thickness, scanning speed, (Seeram, Berland, Curry)**

370. **(C)** Raw data contains the values of detector from all views and rays within a scan. Raw data would be convolved with filters and then projected as image data. **raw data, convolution filters, image data (Berland, Seeram, Haaga, Carlton, Bushberg, Curry)**

371. **(B)** Window level is the central value in a range gray shades use to display the image . **window level, gray scale (Carlton, Seeram, Berland, Bushong, Bushberg, Lee)**

372. **(D)** Decreasing section thickness will increase resolution, decrease voxel size, and increase reconstruction time. **section thickness, resolution, voxel, scan time (Berland, Bushberg, Seeram, Carlton, Bushong, Hendee)**

373. **(A)** +1,000 is within the CT or Hounsfield unit range for bone. **CT numbers, Hounsfield numbers (Seeram, Bushberg, Berland, Wolbarst, Bushong, Carlton, Curry, Hendee)**

374. **(C)** CT numbers between -150 and +150 would be assigned gray values for a 300 WW and 0 WL. **window width, window level, CT numbers (Seeram, Carlton, Bushong, Berland )**

375. **(D)** If a window width of 200 and a window level of +40 is selected, the gray scale range would be -60 to +140, therefore CT numbers below -60 would be black. **window width, window level, CT numbers (Seeram, Carlton, Bushong, Berland )**

376. **(B)** A voxel represents a volume element. **voxel, volume element (Seeram, Berland, Carlton, Curry, Bushberg, Wolbarst)**

377. **(C)** An algorithm is a series of mathematical calculations. **algorithm (Wolbarst, Carlton, Bushberg, Seeram, Bushong)**

378. **(D)** A smaller field of view results in less tissue represented per voxel, spatial resolution is increased, and the display image is magnified. **matrix, field of view, spatial resolution, magnification (Berland, Bushberg, Hendee)**

379. **(A)** The laser camera system creates less scattered light which produces superior high contrast film images. Laser cameras do not require a photographic focusing lens. Laser systems are more expensive than multiformat systems. **laser camera, multiformat camera (Bushberg, KU, Carlton, Seeram)**

380. **(A)** The pixel values in the image data determine the intensity of the laser beam in a laser camera. **laser camera (Bushberg, Carlton, Kuni)**

381. **(A)** Photographic film is used in computed tomography to record the image. Photographic film only needs a single emulsion because brightness and exposure time can be easily adjusted. **photographic film, single emulsion (Berland, Carlton, Bushong)**

382. **(B)** The equation is solved by multiplying the section thickness 5mm by the pixel size 0.75mm$^2$. Remember the pixel is two dimensional and the voxel is three dimensional, therefore the voxel size equals 5mm x 0.75mm x 0.75mm = 2.81$^3$. **voxel size (Bushong, Carlton, Berland)**

383. **(C)** Blood and muscle are represented by CT or Hounsfield numbers above 0. Water is 0 on both the CT and Hounsfield scales. **CT numbers, Hounsfield numbers (Seeram, Bushberg, Berland, Wolbarst, Bushong, Carlton, Curry, Hendee)**

384. **(D)** A region of interest measurement of CT data mean attenuation of CT numbers, standard deviation of CT numbers which is the amount of CT number variation within a region. The ROI function is selected by the technologist and applied to an area of pixels on the monitor. The ROI can be elliptical, circular or square in shape. **region of interest, ROI (Seeram, Berland, Carlton, Brooker, Haaga)**

385. **(C)** A histogram provides a graphic presentation of the distribution of CT numbers and the amplitude of the relative number of points within a particular region of interest. **histogram, region of interest (Berland, Seeram)**

386. **(C)** Helical/spiral data is collected as the patient is moved through the scan field as the x-ray tube simultaneously rotates around the patient. The Helical/spiral data must be changed to axial or planar data. If the data were reconstructed at this point motion artifacts would be present. A sliding filter is applied to the Helical/spiral data to compensate for the continuous transport of the patient. Linear interpolation is the simplest form used to change Helical/spiral data into planar data. **linear interpolation, helical/spiral CT (Picker, Toshiba, Seeram, Bushberg)**

387. **(D)** Volume averaging, artifacts, and mixed attenuated lesions are causes of CT number variances within a region of interest measurement. **volume averaging, artifacts, mixed attenuated lesions, ROI (Berland, Seeram, Carlton, Bushong, Bushberg, Wolbarst)**

388. **(A)** Retrospective reconstructions or secondary reconstructions are performed from the raw data after the initial reconstruction takes place. **retrospective reconstruction, raw data (Berland, Seeram, Curry, Carlton, Bushberg)**

389. **(A)** Magnification of the image enlarges the information from one pixel and displays it over several pixels. The magnification of the image is the manipulation of image data only. Targeted reconstructed images are superior to magnification of an image. **magnification, targeting (Berland, Seeram, Carlton, Bushong)**

390. **(D)** Inter scan delay (ISD) is the delay from section to section in conventional CT due to the start-stop action of the tube and the detector assembly, start-stop action associated with patient breathing, and the time it takes for the table to move from one point to another. **inter scan delay (Seeram, Berland, Brooker, Picker, Toshiba)**

# Image Quality                                    *(#391-423)*

391. **(D)** The signal to noise ratio increases (thus decreasing noise) as mAs is increased, section thickness in increased (widened), and detection efficiency is increased. **noise, signal to noise ratio, detectors, section thickness (Berland, Wolbarst, Carlton, Hendee, Bushong, Bushberg)**

392. **(A)** Increasing mAs will increase the quantity of photons reaching the detectors, thus compensating to avoid quantum noise when performing thin section computed tomography. **noise, section thickness (Berland, Seeram)**

393. **(B)** Increasing matrix size, decreases pixel size which decreases partial volume effect therefore, spatial resolution is increased. Enlarging the focal spot and decreasing the number of projections, decreases spatial resolution. **matrix size, spatial resolution (Curry, Berland, Seeram, Bushberg, Carlton)**

394. **(C)** Linearity defines the relationship of CT numbers to the linear attenuation coefficients of objects imaged. **linearity, CT numbers (Seeram, Berland, Carlton, Bushberg)**

395. **(B)** An increase in section thickness will decrease noise if the technical factors remain unchanged. **section thickness, noise (Berland, Seeram, Curry, Bushberg)**

396. **(D)** Quantum noise, structural noise, and electronic noise are all types of noise that can effect resolution of a CT image. **noise, image degradation (Berland, Seeram, Curry, Wolbarst, Bushberg)**

397. **(C)** A high spatial frequency or high pass algorithm is a bone or edge enhancing algorithm. The high pass algorithm would increase image noise, increase edge enhancement, and decrease contrast resolution and low contrast detectibility of lesions within the organs of the abdomen. **high spatial frequency algorithm, CT abdomen (Seeram, Berland, Haaga, Webb)**

398. **(B)** Contrast resolution can be defined as the ability to display an image of a large object that is only slightly different in density from its surroundings. **contrast resolution (Seeram, Berland, Curry, Bushberg)**

399. **(B)** CT contrast resolution is superior than that of conventional screen-film radiography. CT can detect density differences of 0.25%-0.50% compared to 10% that screen-film radiography can detect. Conventional radiography spatial resolution is superior than that of computed tomography. **contrast resolution, spatial resolution (Bushberg, Seeram, Berland, Carlton, Bushong)**

400. **(B)** The limiting resolution of a CT scanner of 8 line pairs per centimeter is solved is equal to the reciprocal of the spatial frequency. 1/8 lp/cm = 10/8 lp/mm = 1.25 lp/mm. The answer 1.25 must be divided by 2, or halved to reduce line pair. The size of the object that can be resolved is 0.6mm. **CT scanner resolving power, line pairs/centimeter (Seeram, Bushong, Berland, Curry)**

401. **(C)** A water phantom calibration test determines the spatial uniformity and noise performance of a CT scanner. **quality assurance, water calibration test (Seeram, Berland)**

402. **(A)** The CT number range within the water phantom should be -3 to +3 range from the attenuation value of water for

a CT scanner to pass this test. **quality assurance, water calibration test (Seeram, Hendee)**

403. **(A)** Spatial resolution refers to resolution coordinates in the x and y imaging planes. **spatial resolution (Wolbarst, Bushberg, Seeram)**

404. **(A)** The lung and inner ear are regions of high contrast which require viewing with a relatively wide window width. **window width (Berland, Seeram, Carlton, Bushong)**

405. **(C)** Quantum noise is decreased by increasing section thickness because more photons become available to provide information. Quantum noise is increased when mAs or kVp are decreased because the quantity of photons available decreases. **noise, section thickness (Berland, Seeram)**

406. **(A)** A CT water calibration should be done daily. **quality assurance, water calibration test (Seeram, Berland)**

407. **(B)** Pitch is a term that describes the extension of a helix. If pitch increases, patient dose decreases because the area being scanned will be covered in a shorter time period than that of a pitch of 1 (section thickness=table speed mm/second. **pitch, helical/spiral CT (Picker, Toshiba, Bushberg, Seeram)**

408. **(C)** Applying a filter to the back projection reconstruction method changes the attenuation profiles which eliminates the streak and star artifacts that are associated with back projection reconstruction. **back projection reconstruction, filtered back projection reconstruction (Seeram, Berland, Curry, Carlton, Wolbarst, Bushberg)**

409. **(C)** Spatial resolution is defined as the ability to distinguish details in objects of different densities a small distance apart especially in high density regions. **spatial resolution (Seeram, Berland, Curry, Carlton, Wolbarst, Bushberg)**

410. **(D)** Low contrast detectibility is a term used to describe contrast resolution. **contrast resolution, low con-**

trast detectibility **(Seeram, Berland, Curry, Bushberg)**

411. **(D)** Soft tissue resolution can be maximized by a low spatial frequency or low pass algorithm, utilization of narrow window widths, and low window levels. A low pass algorithm is a standard algorithm that is designed to enhance soft tissue resolution. **contrast resolution, soft tissue resolution (Seeram, Berland, Picker)**

412. **(C)** CT usually uses relatively high kV ranges (120-140). At these high ranges the photoelectric effect is only a minor contributor of attenuation. Compton scattering is the primary type of interaction that contributes to the subject contrast in the image. **Compton scattering, photoelectric effect (Bushberg, Carlton, Wolbarst, Bushong, Curry)**

413. **(A)** The modular transfer function is a curve that results from plotting spatial frequency against a modular transfer function. The MTF is the most commonly used descriptor for quantifying spatial resolution. **(Seeram, Berland, Bushong)**

414. **(B)** Patient dose increases are a direct result of increases of scanning technical factors. Increasing the technical factors produces an increase in the number of photons that reach the detector. This directly results in an increased detector signal which provides more information for the formation of the image hence, noise decreases. **patient dose, noise (Seeram, Berland, Wolbarst, Bushberg, Curry)**

415. **(A)** The signal to noise ratio is the primary factor that determines the degree of contrast resolution that a CT system is capable of producing. **signal to noise ratio, contrast resolution (Seeram, Berland, Wolbarst, Bushberg, Carlton)**

416. **(C)** A decrease in scanning technical factors, decreases the amount of photons that reach the detector. This results in a decrease in patient dose which decreases low contrast resolution. **contrast resolution (Seeram, Berland, Bushberg, Curry)**

417. **(A)** If kVp, mA, and time remain constant an increase of section thickness from 5mm to 10mm doubles the

number of detected x-ray photons. **section thickness (Bushberg, Seeram, Berland)**

418. **(A)** Dynamic scanning requires a decrease in technical factors to avoid tube heating problems. The decrease in technical factors decrease the number of photons reaching the detector which decreases the detector signal and increases quantum noise. **quantum noise, noise (Seeram, Berland, Bushberg, Curry)**

419. **(A)** The size of the row of holes that can be clearly visualized from a test pattern determines the performance of the CT scanner relative to low contrast resolution. The smaller the size of the row of holes that can be clearly visualized the better the performance of the scanner. **contrast resolution, quality assurance (Seeram, Berland, Bushberg, Wolbarst)**

420. **(D)** Application of a high spatial frequency algorithm, thin section thickness (1-3mm), and a small field of view maximizes spatial resolution for CT of the temporal bones. **spatial resolution, temporal bones (Seeram, Berland, Som, Haaga)**

421. **(D)** The multi scan average dose (MSAD) represents the average dose a patient a receives during a series of scans. The MSAD also represents the dose that the center section receives for a series of scans. If the table index is decreased the MSAD increases. **multi scan average dose (MSAD) (Seeram, Berland, Behrman)**

422. **(D)** The computed tomography dose index (CTDI) is defined as the area of one dose profile divided by the section thickness for contiguous sections. The CTDI of a CT scanner is measured with an ionization chamber. The MSAD can be calculated from the CTDI, if table index equals section thickness MSAD equals CTDI. **computed tomography dose index (CTDI) (Seeram, Behrman, Berland)**

423. **(C)** Oversampling is accomplished by aligning the central axis of rotation with a point that is 1/4 the width of the detector. **oversampling, number of projections (Bushberg, Wolbarst, Seeram)**

## Artifacts                                      (#424-450)

424. **(B)**  Ring artifacts are produced by tube-detector misalignment in third generation rotate-rotate geometry scanners. **rotate-rotate, third generation scanners, ring artifacts (Bushberg, Seeram, Berland, Brooker, Curry)**

425. **(D)**  Low density streaks adjacent to high density structures, general CT number shift, and cupping artifacts are all related to beam hardening. **beam hardening effect (Seeram, Berland, Bushberg, Curry)**

426. **(C)**  A cupping artifact is a result of the body hardening the beam lowering the attenuation values in the center of the image. **beam hardening, cupping artifact (Seeram, Berland, Bushberg, Wolbarst)**

427. **(A)**  A capping artifact arises when the computer overcorrects for beam hardening. **beam hardening, capping artifact (Seeram, Berland, Bushberg)**

428. **(D)**  Star artifacts are caused by high density objects in the patient such as dental fillings, surgical clips etc. **star artifacts (Seeram, Berland, Wolbarst, Bushberg)**

429. **(A)**  Streak artifacts arise from patient motion because the reconstruction algorithms inability to compensate for the inconsistencies of voxel attenuations from the edge of a moving part. **motion artifacts (Seeram, Berland, Bushberg, Curry)**

430. **(C)**  Partial volume artifacts can be described as bands or streaks across an area due to two or more attenuation values occupying a single pixel. **partial volume artifacts (Seeram, Berland, Bushberg, Wolbarst, Haaga)**

431. **(A)**  The dynamic range is the range of x-ray intensities that a detector receives and responds to linearly. The larger the dynamic range the better the response. **dynamic range, CT numbers, artifacts (Haaga, Seeram, Berland)**

432. **(A)**  Added filtration near the x-ray tube and the use of beam hardening corrections will reduce beam hardening effect. **beam hardening, filtration, algorithms (Berland, Seeram, Bushberg, Wolbarst, Curry)**

433. **(B)** Edge gradient artifacts cause streaking artifacts which is oriented tangentially to a flat surface having a high spatial frequency. **edge gradient artifacts (Berland, Seeram)**

434. **(A)** A decrease in section thickness would also require an increase in mAs to maintain the same signal to noise performance of the scanner. To minimize the partial volume effect both of the factors would have to be adjusted. **partial volume effect, signal to noise ratio (Seeram, Berland, Bushberg, Haaga)**

435. **(D)** Motion artifacts can be minimized for fourth generation scanners by increasing scan time. The increase in scan time must be used to perform an overscan. **overscan, fourth generation geometry (Berland)**

436. **(D)** Thoracotomy tubes, a patient's arms, and ventilator tubing can produce beam hardening which results in out of field artifacts. **beam hardening effect, out of field artifacts (Seeram, Berland, Bushberg, Brooker)**

437. **(D)** The edge gradient effect, nonlinear partial volume effect, and the beam hardening effect contribute to the formation of artifacts from structures containing metal. **metallic artifacts (Berland, Seeram, Brooker, Haaga, Bushberg)**

438. **(A)** The "bow tie" filter minimizes beam hardening artifacts and reduces scatter radiation. **beam filtration, filters (Berland, Carlton)**

439. **(B)** An interpolation algorithm is applied to the raw data before the reconstruction process begins. This is known as z-axis weighting of spiral data and is designed to compensate for the continuous patient transport during helical/spiral scanning. **interpolation, helical/spiral CT (Picker, Toshiba, Seeram, Bushberg)**

440. **(A)** Patient motion, body movement or inconsistent breathing can result in misregistration of the image and can produce step-like contours which can resemble fractures on the three dimensional reconstructed image. **3D reconstruction, patient motion, image misregistration (Seeram, Berland, Picker, Bushberg, Brooker)**

441. **(D)** Image ghosting, image blurring, and streak artifacts can result from patient motion during a scan. **motion artifacts (Seeram, Berland, Bushberg, Brooker, Haaga)**

442. **(A)** Ailiasing artifacts arise from high frequency areas when too few samples or views are obtained. **ailiasing artifacts (Berland, Seeram, Bushberg, Wolbarst)**

443. **(B)** Ring artifacts are a characteristic of third generation scanners. If a detector has an offset or gain difference from the other detectors, a circular artifact will be present on the image. The solution to correct the problem is recalibrating the detector gain. **ring artifacts, detector gain (Seeram, Berland, Bushberg, Curry)**

444. **(B)** When sampling is insufficient, streak artifacts may arise on the scanogram. **sample ailiasing, scanogram (Berland, Seeram)**

445. **(B)** Annular ring artifacts typical of third generation scanners are caused by one detector being out of calibration. The closer the faulty detector is to the center of the scanning beam, the smaller the diameter of the artifact. **artifacts, computed tomography generation configurations (Berland, Bushberg)**

446. **(D)** Biopsy needles, bone to soft tissue interfaces, and cracks in the scanning table all result in edge gradient artifacts. **edge gradient artifacts (Berland, Seeram, Bushberg, Curry)**

447. **(A)** A decrease in scan time will reduce patient motion artifacts. **motion artifacts (Berland, Seeram, Brooker, Curry)**

448. **(B)** Vaporization of the anode and filament is responsible for tube arching. Tube arching artifacts result in large bizarre bands or streaks on the image. **tube arching, artifacts (Berland, Carlton, Bushong)**

449. **(D)** Missing sections from a stack of sections, beam hardening artifacts, and patient motion degrade three dimensional reconstructed images. **three dimensional images, image degradation (Seeram, Berland, Bushberg)**

450. **(A)** Artifacts from scatter radiation mimic beam hardening artifacts. Scatter artifacts can be minimized by post patient collimation and by placing a set of secondary detectors adjacent to the primary detectors but outside the range of primary radiation. **scatter radiation, artifacts (Bushberg, Berland, Seeram, Wolbarst)**

# Patient Care (#1 - #30)

1. Which portion of the adult sternum is compressed during cardiopulmonary resuscitation?

    ___ a.  upper half

    ___ b.  lower half

    ___ c.  entire surface

    ___ d.  xiphoid process

2. Which of the following is the proper way to administer nitroglycerin to a patient who is experiencing angina pectoris?

    ___ a.  orally

    ___ b.  sublingually

    ___ c.  intramuscularly

    ___ d.  intravenously

3. Which of the following routes of drug administration would result in the fastest response?

    ___ a.  orally

    ___ b.  subcutaneously

    ___ c.  intramuscularly

    ___ d.  intravenously

4. What type of drug is Demerol?

    ___ a.  analgesic

    ___ b.  antipyretic

    ___ c.  antianxiety agent

    ___ d.  local anesthetic

5. A patient's blood pressure is 120/90. What does the figure 120 represent?

___ a. pressure of ventricular relaxation

___ b. systolic pressure

___ c. diastolic pressure

___ d. low blood pressure

6. If a patient convulses in the CT department, the technologist should do which of the following?

___ a. insert a padded tongue blade

___ b. restrain the patient

___ c. prevent injury to the patient

___ d. put the patient on the floor

7. Which of the following terms would best define air in the pleural space?

___ a. pleural effusion

___ b. atelectasis

___ c. hemothorax

___ d. pneumothorax

8. Which of the following describes rapid, irregular, ineffective twitches of the ventricles?

___ a. ventricular regurgitation

___ b. ventricular palpitations

___ c. ventricular arrythmia

___ d. ventricular fibrillation

9. Which of the following is the definition for the term dyspnea?

___ a. excess fluid in body tissue

___ b. rapid heart rate

___ c. abnormal blood flow

___ d. difficulty breathing

10. Which of the following is the technical term for a heart attack?

    ___ a.  dyspnea

    ___ b.  angina pectoris

    ___ c.  myocardial infarction

    ___ d.  ataxia

11. A patient whose skin has a bluish tinge due to a lack of oxygen in his or her blood is suffering fron what condition?

    ___ a.  pallor

    ___ b.  edema

    ___ c.  diaphoresis

    ___ d.  cyanosis

12. What type of shock can result from a severe reaction to the contrast media used in radiographic exams?

    ___ a.  hypovolemic

    ___ b.  septic

    ___ c.  cardiogenic

    ___ d.  anaphylatic

13. What type of patient reaction to an injection of water-soluble iodine contrast usually does not require treatment?

    ___ a.  metallic taste on injection

    ___ b.  chest pain

    ___ c.  dyspnea

    ___ d.  tachycardia

14. Which of the following is typically associated with shock?

    ___ a.  flushed face

    ___ b.  decreasing blood pressure

    ___ c.  decreasing pulse rate

    ___ d.  fever

15. In working with a patient, which of the following would be the first priority for attention?

___ a. treating shock

___ b. controlling bleeding

___ c. splinting a fractured extremity

___ d. providing an open airway

16. Why is anaphylactic shock the type of shock most often seen in the CT scanning area?

___ a. it is caused by contrast media use

___ b. most CT patients are very weak

___ c. its effects are enhanced by radiation

___ d. many CT patients are hypertensive

17. Which of the following is the more toxic cation that is incorporated into the organic ionic contrast media?

___ a. sodium

___ b. meglumine

___ c. iodine

___ d. calcium

18. While scanning a patient with chest-tube drainage, which of the following actions should be taken?

___ a. clamp drainage tube

___ b. keep drainage system below chest

___ c. raise drainage system above chest

___ d. turn pump off during the exam

19. What is the term that indicates a telescoping of the bowel into itself?

___ a. intussusception

___ b. volvulus

___ c. atresia

___ d. herniation

20. Which of the following is usually a complication of esophageal varices?

___ a.  hiatal hernia

___ b.  portal venous hypertension

___ c.  biliary atresia

___ d.  gastric distension

21. Which of the following describes a sudden distant cerebral neurologic deficit of presumed vascular origin usually lasting a few minutes?

___ a.  transient ischemic attack (TIA)

___ b.  steady progressive from onset (SPO)

___ c.  single catastrophic episode (SCE)

___ d.  occlusive vascular disease (OVD)

22. Which of the following refers to a constriction or narrowing of a blood vessel?

___ a.  stenosis

___ b.  thrombosis

___ c.  edema

___ d.  aneurysm

23. A diabetic patient whose skin is dry and has a fruity odor on their breath is a classic example of which situation?

___ a.  drunkenness

___ b.  insulin shock

___ c.  diabetes

___ d.  diabetic coma

24. What is the most severe form of convulsive seizure?

___ a.  petit mal

___ b.  partial

___ c.  grand mal

___ d.  epileptic

25. What are the required settings for constant flow injectors?

    ___ a. pressure and time

    ___ b. flow rate and time

    ___ c. volume and pressure

    ___ d. flow rate and volume

26. Into what positions should a patient be moved to avoid aspiration of vomitus?

    1. lateral recumbent
    2. sitting
    3. supine

    ___ a. 1 & 2 only

    ___ b. 1 & 3 only

    ___ c. 2 & 3 only

    ___ d. 1, 2, & 3

27. How long is the injection time for 12 ml of contrast media delivered at 2.5 ml/sec?

    ___ a. 0.2 sec

    ___ b. 2.5 sec

    ___ c. 4.8 sec

    ___ d. 30 sec

28. What type of drug should be considered for a patient who complains of having "tongue thickness"?

    ___ a. antihistamine

    ___ b. sedative

    ___ c. anesthetic

    ___ d. anticoagulant

29. How is the measurement of the flow rate of an automatic contrast injector determined?

    ___ a. contrast amount delivered per unit time

    ___ b. heating device

    ___ c. contrast volume times contrast size

    ___ d. syringe size

30. How long does it take for interstitial diffusion of contrast media to occur within the body tissues after beginning an injection?

   \_\_ a. less than 5 seconds

   \_\_ b. 30 seconds

   \_\_ c. 2 - 4 minutes

   \_\_ d. more than 5 minutes

# Imaging Procedures (#31-105)

## Head (#31-45)

31. Which of the following would be visualized on a coronal CT scan of the head?

    1.  sellar floor
    2.  suprasellar cistern
    3.  pituitary gland thickness

    ___ a.  1 and 2
    ___ b.  1 and 3
    ___ c.  2 and 3
    ___ d.  1, 2, & 3

32. Which of the following describes the basal ganglia of the brain?

    ___ a.  gray matter regions of the cerebrum
    ___ b.  a band of white fibers that connects the two cerebral hemispheres
    ___ c.  located in the brainstem
    ___ d.  the long narrow cerebrospinal fluid channel that descends through the midbrain

33. What term is used to describe the computed tomography appearance of an intracerebral hemorrhage as a result of a higher CT number of the hemorrhage as compared to normal brain tissue?

    ___ a.  hyperdense
    ___ b.  isodense
    ___ c.  hypodense
    ___ d.  mass effect

34. Which of the following are causes of an spontaneous hemor-rhages in the brain?

    1. hypertension
    2. rupture of an aneurysm
    3. bleeding from a arteriovenous malformation

    ___ a.  1 only

    ___ b.  2 only

    ___ c.  3 only

    ___ d.  1, 2, & 3

35. What patient position is used for coronal exams of the head?

    1. supine, head extended
    2. prone, head extended
    3. supine, routine head position

    ___ a.  1

    ___ b.  2

    ___ c.  3

    ___ d.  1 & 2

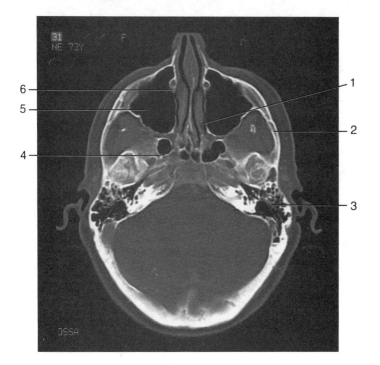

*Figure PT 1*

36. Which of the following is illustrated by #1 in Figure PT 1?

    ___ a.  inferior nasal concha

    ___ b.  vomer

    ___ c.  nasal septum

    ___ d.  nasolacrimal duct

37. Which of the following is illustrated by #5 in Figure PT 1?

    ___ a.  ethmoid sinus

    ___ b.  sphenoid sinus

    ___ c.  maxillary sinus

    ___ d.  frontal sinus

38. Which of the following is illustrated by #3 in Figure PT 1?

    ___ a.  temporal sinus

    ___ b.  mastoid air cells

    ___ c.  ethmoid sinus

    ___ d.  external auditory meatus

39. Which of the following are classifications of subdural hematomas?

   1.  acute

   2.  subacute

   3.  chronic

      __  a.  1 and 2

      __  b.  1 and 3

      __  c.  2 and 3

      __  d.  1, 2, & 3

40. Which of the following statements are true regarding coronal
computed tomography examination of the sinuses?

   1.  the scan extent is from the beginning of the frontal sinus
through the entire sphenoid sinus

   2.  1mm to 5mm coronal sections should be acquired through
the osteomeatal complex

   3.  the hard palate is perpendicular to the scan beam

      __  a.  1 and 2

      __  b.  1 and 3

      __  c.  2 and 3

      __  d.  1, 2, & 3

41. Which of the following techniques could the computed to-
mographer utilize to minimize patient motion when performing a CT examination of the head?

   1.  taping across the head and chin

   2.  placing of sponges on both sides of the head

   3.  Diazepam sedation

      __  a.  1 and 2

      __  b.  1 and 3

      __  c.  2 and 3

      __  d.  1, 2, & 3

42. Which of the following is the angle that is utilized for routine axial sections of the brain?

1. parallel to the orbitomeatal line
2. 10-20 degrees to the orbitomeatal line
3. 30-40 degrees to the orbitomeatal line

___ a. 1 only

___ b. 2 only

___ c. 3 only

___ d. 1,2,& 3

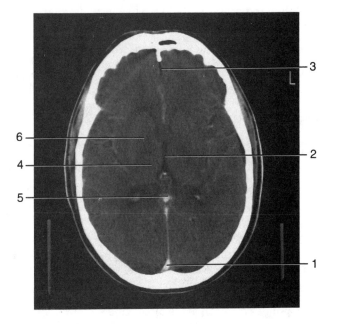

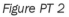
*Figure PT 2*

43. Which of the following is illustrated by #1 on the contrast enhanced image of the head Figure PT 2?

___ a. basilar artery

___ b. superior sagittal sinus

___ c. fourth ventricle

___ d. choroid plexus

44. Which of the following illustrated by #3 on the contrast enhanced image of the head Figure PT 2?

___ a.  falx cerebri

___ b.  septum pellucidum

___ c.  third ventricle

___ d.  sylvian fissure

45. Which of the following is illustrated by #4 on the contrast enhanced image of the brain Figure PT 2?

___ a.  caudate nucleus

___ b.  corpus callosum

___ c.  thalamus

___ d.  cerebral peduncle

# Neck                                                    (#46-48)

46. What position should the patient's upper extremities be positioned for routine CT scanning of the neck?

___ a.  the shoulders should be pulled down as far as possible and the arms placed at the sides

___ b.  the shoulders are extended and the arms are raised above the head

___ c.  the shoulders should be relaxed and the arms are placed on top of the body

___ d.  the shoulders are rolled forward and the arms are placed at the sides

47. What are the best breathing instructions for the patient during an exam of the larynx?

___ a.  deep inspiration and suspend during each scan

___ b.  exhalation and suspend breathing during each scan

___ c.  suspend respiration and swallowing the same during each scan

___ d.  quiet respiration without swallowing during each scan

48. Which of the following are reasons intravenous contrast media would be used for CT scanning of the neck?

  1. differentiate small nodes from vessels
  2. determine relationship between a mass to vessels
  3. trauma to the larynx

  ___ a. 1 and 2
  ___ b. 1 and 3
  ___ c. 2 and 3
  ___ d. 1, 2, & 3

# Spine                                              (#49-59)

49. What is the most common section orientation for routine CT scanning of the lumbar spine?

  ___ a. perpendicular to the plane of the intervertebral disc space
  ___ b. parallel to the plane of the intervertebral disc space
  ___ c. 45 degree oblique to the plane of the intervertebral disc space
  ___ d. 70 degree oblique to the plane of the intervertebral disc space

50. In what position should a patient's head be placed for post myelography CT of the spine?

  ___ a. lower than the body
  ___ b. rotated laterally from the body
  ___ c. elevated higher than the body
  ___ d. parallel to the body

51. What is the most common scan extent for a routine conventional CT examination of the lumbar spine?

  ___ a. from the mid body of L3 to the top of S1
  ___ b. from the top of L1 to the top of S1
  ___ c. from the mid body of L3 to the end of the sacrum
  ___ d. from the mid body of L2 to the end of L5

52. What is the primary reason for scanning a patient in the prone position for a post myelogram CT of the spine?

    __ a. minimizes the effects of the intrathecal contrast layering or pooling

    __ b. prevents the contrast from mixing with the cerebrospinal fluid

    __ c. it is more comfortable for the patient

    __ d. decreases the length of scan time

53. Which of the following contrast media would best differentiate between scar and recurrent disc herniation in the lumbar spine?

    __ a. water-based intrathecal contrast

    __ b. oily-based intrathecal contrast

    __ c. intravenous contrast

    __ d. negative (air) contrast

54. Which of the following positions may be used to decrease lordosis of the lumbar spine?

    __ a. supine, thighs extended

    __ b. prone, thighs extended

    __ c. supine, thighs flexed

    __ d. prone, thighs flexed

55. Which of the following are normal variants that can confuse a technologist when locating a starting and ending point for a CT examination of the lumbar spine?

1. sacralization of the L5 vertebral body
2. a rib bearing lumbar vertebrae
3. absence of a lumbar vertebrae

    __ a. 1 only

    __ b. 2 only

    __ c. 3 only

    __ d. 1, 2, & 3

56. Which of the following conditions would coronal reconstructions of the spine be most useful?

   1. determining spinal fusion integrity
   2. medial and lateral fracture fragment displacements
   3. determining the extent of spinal cord encroachment of posterior displaced fracture fragments

   ___ a. 1 and 2
   ___ b. 1 and 3
   ___ c. 2 and 3
   ___ d. 1, 2, & 3

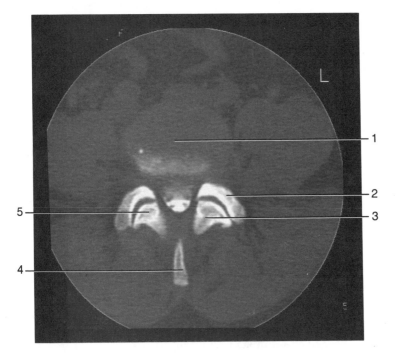

*Figure PT 3*

57. Which of the following is illustrated by #2 in Figure PT 3?

   ___ a. transverse process
   ___ b. inferior articular process
   ___ c. superior articular process
   ___ d. pedicle

58. Which of the following is illustrated by #3 in Figure PT 3?

___ a.   transverse process

___ b.   inferior articular process

___ c.   superior articular process

___ d.   pedicle

59. Which of the following is illustrated by #1 in Figure PT 3?

___ a.   spinal canal

___ b.   vertebral body

___ c.   intervertebral disc

___ d.   abdominal aorta

## Chest                                                            (#60-74)

60. What term is used to describe a left mediastinal space bounded anteriorly, superiorly, and posteriorly by the ascending aorta, bounded inferiorly by the left pulmonary artery, and bounded medially by the lower trachea and proximal left main bronchus?

___ a.   hilum

___ b.   aorticopulmonary window

___ c.   pleural space

___ d.   carina

61. Which of the following levels are usually dynamically scanned when a dissecting thoracic aneurysm is suspected?

1.   at the aortic arch
2.   at the proximal aortic root and proximal descending aorta at the level of the right pulmonary artery
3.   at the distal descending thoracic aorta

___ a.   1 and 2

___ b.   1 and 3

___ c.   2 and 3

___ d.   1, 2, & 3

62. Which of the following occurs when a high resolution technique is used for a CT scan of the lungs?

    1. image smoothing is reduced
    2. spatial resolution is increased
    3. visible image noise decreases

        ___ a.  1 and 2
        ___ b.  1 and 3
        ___ c.  2 and 3
        ___ d.  1, 2, & 3

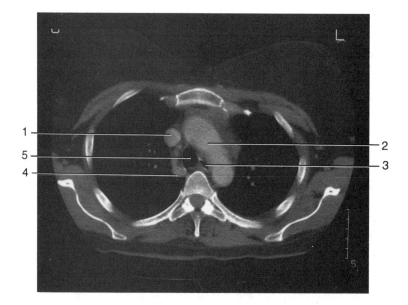

Figure PT 4

63. Which of the following is illustrated by #2 in Figure PT 4?

    ___ a.  superior vena cava
    ___ b.  left atrium
    ___ c.  left ventricle
    ___ d.  aortic arch

64. Which of the following is illustrated by #5 in Figure PT 4?

   __ a. trachea

   __ b. esophagus

   __ c. main stem bronchus

   __ d. thyroid gland

65. Which of the following is illustrated by #1 in Figure PT 4?

   __ a. superior vena cava

   __ b. right pulmonary artery

   __ c. azygos vein

   __ d. inferior vena cava

66. What is the best section thickness for a high resolution CT scan of the lungs?

   __ a. 1mm to 2mm

   __ b. 3mm to 5mm

   __ c. 8mm to 10mm

   __ d. 12mm to 15mm

67. Which of the following positions may help to distinguish the separation of fluids or fluid levels in the chest?

1. prone
2. right lateral decubitus
3. left lateral decubitus

   __ a. 1 and 2

   __ b. 1 and 3

   __ c. 2 and 3

   __ d. 1, 2, & 3

68. In what phase of respiration should conventional CT scans of the mediastinum be performed?

   __ a. end tidal volume

   __ b. suspended expiration

   __ c. suspended inspiration

   __ d. rapid breathing

69. What is the most common scout view obtained for a CT examination of the chest?

___ a. AP

___ b. lateral

___ c. oblique

___ d. decubitus

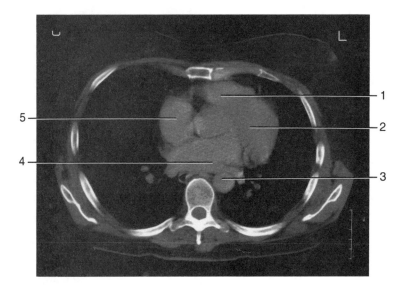

*Figure PT 5*

70. Which of the following is illustrated by #5 in Figure PT 5?

___ a. superior vena cava

___ b. right atrium

___ c. right ventricle

___ d. acending aorta

71. Which of the following is illustrated by #3 in Figure PT 5?

___ a. inferior vena cava

___ b. azygos vein

___ c. descending aorta

___ d. superior vena cava

72. Which of the following is illustrated by #4 in Figure PT 5?

___ a. right atrium

___ b. right ventricle

___ c. left atrium

___ d. left ventricle

73. Which of the following positions may be used for better demonstration of the posterior lung bases?

___ a. supine

___ b. prone

___ c. lateral decubitus

___ d. 45 degree oblique

74. Which of the following combinations of section thickness and table incrementations would produce the most accurate 3D image reformations of blood vessels of the thorax?

___ a. 5mm section thickness, 5mm table incrementation

___ b. 5mm section thickness, 10mm table incrementation

___ c. 5mm section thickness, 3mm table incrementation

___ d. 10mm section thickness, 10mm table incrementation

# Abdomen (#75-89)

75. Which of the following provides optimal liver lesion detection following the introduction of contrast media?

1. scanning prior to the equilibrium phase
2. scanning during the equilibrium phase
3. scanning after the equilibrium phase

___ a. 1 only

___ b. 2 only

___ c. 3 only

___ d. 1, 2, & 3

76. What is the total volume of an abdomen scanned utilizing the helical/spiral acquisition method if the scan time is 1 sec/rota-

tion, total scanning time is 30 seconds, section thickness is 10mm, and tabletop speed is 10mm/sec?

___ a. 100mm

___ b. 200mm

___ c. 300mm

___ d. 400mm

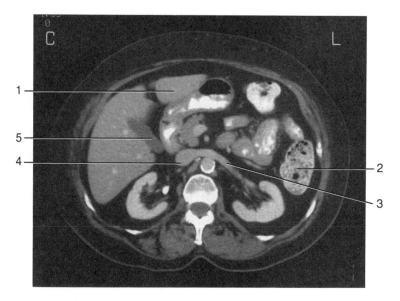

*Figure PT 6*

77. Which of the following is illustrated by #2 in Figure PT 6?

___ a. jejunum

___ b. acending colon

___ c. descending colon

___ d. cecum

78. Which of the following is illustrated by #3 in Figure PT 6?

___ a. left renal artery

___ b. left renal vein

___ c. adrenal gland

___ d. inferior venal cava

79. Which of the following is illustrated by #1 in Figure PT 6?

    __ a.  pancreas

    __ b.  left lateral lobe of the liver

    __ c.  gallbladder

    __ d.  transverse colon

80. Which of the following window widths and window levels could be utilized for post scanning filming of the liver?

1. 350/WW, 50/WL
2. 1500/WW, 500/WL
3. 150/WW, 50/WL

    __ a.  1 and 2

    __ b.  1 and 3

    __ c.  2 and 3

    __ d.  1, 2, & 3

81. Which of the following section thicknesses would be the best selection to decrease the possibility of partial volume artifacts occurring when scanning the pancreas?

1. 2mm
2. 5mm
3. 10mm

    __ a.  1 only

    __ b.  2 only

    __ c.  3 only

    __ d.  1, 2, & 3

82. Which of the following algorithms would produce the best low contrast lesion detectability when scanning the abdomen?

1. low spatial frequency algorithm
2. high spatial frequency algorithm
3. bone algorithm

    __ a.  1 only

    __ b.  2 only

    __ c.  3 only

    __ d.  1, 2, & 3

83. Which of the following oral contrast administrations would be used for an exam of the abdomen and pelvis?

1. 300-500 ml given 1-2 hours prior to the exam
2. 300-500 ml given immediately prior to the exam
3. 300-500 ml given at least 4-6 hours prior to the exam

___ a. 1 and 2

___ b. 1 and 3

___ c. 2 and 3

___ d. 1, 2, & 3

84. Which of the following is most likely demonstrated if an ROI measurement is equal to -100?

___ a. air

___ b. bone

___ c. fat

___ d. blood

85. What is the proper breathing technique utilized for a routine abdominal scan?

___ a. suspended inspiration

___ b. suspended expiration

___ c. shallow respiration

___ d. normal respiration

86. Which of the following positions may provide better definition and visualization of the head of the pancreas following the ingestion of oral contrast?

___ a. left decubitus

___ b. right decubitus

___ c. prone

___ d. left posterior oblique

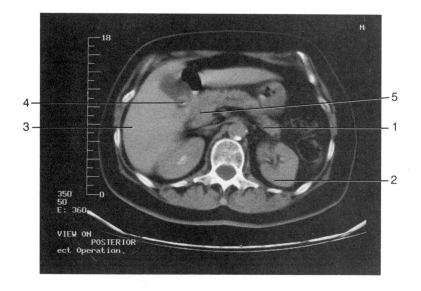

*Figure PT 7*

87. Which of the following is illustrated by #4 in Figure PT 7?

___ a.  gallbladder abscess

___ b.  gallstone

___ c.  calcified portal vein

___ d.  calcified hepatic artery

88. Which of the following is illustrated by #1 in Figure PT 7?

___ a.  duodenum

___ b.  head of the pancreas

___ c.  tail of the pancreas

___ d.  medial lobe of the liver

89. Which of the following is illustrated by #2 in Figure PT 7?

___ a.  left psoas major muscle

___ b.  spleen

___ c.  left kidney

___ d.  splenic flexure of the colon

# Pelvis                                    *(#90-101)*

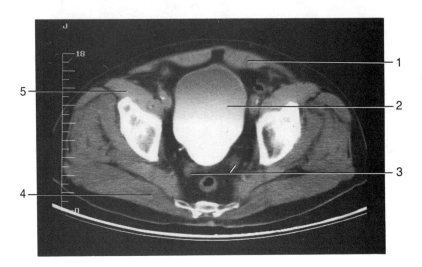

*Figure PT 8*

90. Which of the following is illustrated by #3 in Figure PT 8?

    ___ a.  ureters

    ___ b.  vas deferens

    ___ c.  external iliac arteries

    ___ d.  rectus abdominis muscles

91. Which of the following is illustrated by #2 in Figure PT 8?

    ___ a.  prostate gland

    ___ b.  rectum

    ___ c.  urinary bladder

    ___ d.  intra-abdominal cyst

92. What number illustrates the rectus abdominis muscle in Figure PT 8?

    ___ a.  1

    ___ b.  3

    ___ c.  4

    ___ d.  5

93. Which of the following structures are contained within the true pelvis of the female?

1. uterus
2. vagina
3. ovaries

    ___ a. 1 only

    ___ b. 2 only

    ___ c. 3 only

    ___ d. 1, 2, & 3

94. Which of the following contrast media delivery methods would provide adequate rectosigmoid opacification?

1. 500ml of barium sulfate given orally twelve hours prior to the scan
2. 500ml of barium sulfate introduced rectally prior to the scan
3. 300ml of barium sulfate given orally thirty minutes prior to the scan

    ___ a. 1 and 2

    ___ b. 1 and 3

    ___ c. 2 and 3

    ___ d. 1, 2, & 3

95. What type of scoutview is recommended for a routine CT examination of the pelvis?

    ___ a. AP

    ___ b. lateral

    ___ c. decubitus

    ___ d. oblique

96. Which of the following is the recommended percentage of barium in a barium sulfate suspension utilized in abdominal computed tomography?

    ___ a. 1-3%

    ___ b. 10-20%

    ___ c. 30%

    ___ d. 50%

97. Which of the following is recommended for pelvis exams specifically for examination of the bladder?

      ___ a. the bladder should be filled with urine

      ___ b. the bladder should be emptied just prior to the exam

      ___ c. the bladder should be filled with contrast

      ___ d. the bladder should be kept empty via a catheter

98. Which of the following muscles are found in both the male and female?

  1. levator ani muscle

  2. bulbosponious muscle

  3. transverse perinei muscles

      ___ a. 1 only

      ___ b. 2 only

      ___ c. 3 only

      ___ d. 1, 2, & 3

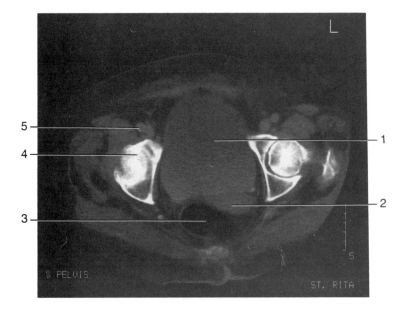

*Figure PT 9*

99. Which of the following is illustrated by #2 in Figure PT 9?

___ a. urinary bladder

___ b. vagina

___ c. uterus

___ d. rectum

100. Which of the following is illustrated by #5 in Figure PT 9?

___ a. femoral artery

___ b. femoral vein

___ c. common iliac artery

___ d. common iliac vein

101. Which of the following is illustrated by #4 in Figure PT 9?

___ a. ischium

___ b. ilium

___ c. head of the femur

___ d. shaft of the femur

## Musculoskeletal                                    *(#102-105)*

102. In which of the following instances is computed tomography superior to magnetic resonance?

    ___ a.  demonstration of ligament injuries

    ___ b.  fractures of complex skeletal regions

    ___ c.  extension of neoplasms into the soft tissues

    ___ d.  demonstration of injuries to labrum

103. Which of the following are reasons that CT would be the imaging modality of choice when imaging trauma to any part of the musculoskeletal system?

1.    minimal positioning maneuvers are required

2.    complex fractures can be thoroughly defined

3.    manipulation of acquired data allows the evaluation of the extent of soft tissue and bony injuries

    ___ a.  1 only

    ___ b.  2 only

    ___ c.  3 only

    ___ d.  1, 2, & 3

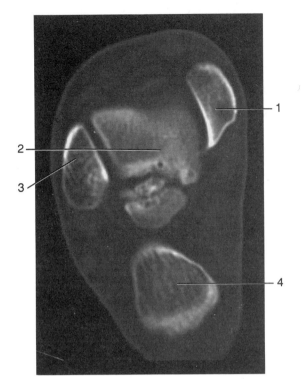

Figure PT 10

104. Which of the following is illustrated by #4 in Figure PT 10?

___ a. talus

___ b. navicular

___ c. cuboid

___ d. calcaneus

105. Which of the following is illustrated by #2 in Figure PT 10?

___ a. talus

___ b. cuboid

___ c. calcaneus

___ d. tibia

# Physics and
# Instrumentation      *(#106-150)*

## System Operation & Components      *(#106-114)*

106. What is the approximate heat unit range for a typical computed tomography x-ray tube anode?

   ___ a.   1.0 - 5.0 hundred
   ___ b.   0.5 - 5.0 thousand
   ___ c.   0.5 - 5.0 million
   ___ d.   10.0 - 25.0 million

107. Which of the following are used in scintillation CT detectors?

1.   gadolinium based ceramics
2.   bismuth germanate
3.   calcium fluoride

   ___ a.   1 and 2
   ___ b.   1 and 3
   ___ c.   2 and 3
   ___ d.   1, 2, & 3

108. How does an array processor increase image processing and display speed?

   ___ a.   by increasing computer processing RAM
   ___ b.   by increasing computer processing ROM
   ___ c.   by performing simultaneous mathematical operations in a parallel fashion
   ___ d.   by decreasing the digital image acquisition data received from the detectors

109. Which of the following are TRUE regarding the highly directional properties of gas filled ionization chamber detectors?

1. it provides a good acceptance angle for primary x-rays
2. it assists in rejecting scatter
3. it eliminates them from use in fourth generation scanners that use a changing alignment between the x-ray beam and detector.

___ a. 1 only
___ b. 2 only
___ c. 3 only
___ d. 1, 2, & 3

110. What is the proper order of descriptions for scan arcs of 220°, 360°, and 400°?

___ a. half scan, full scan, overscan
___ b. full scan, overscan, half scan
___ c. full scan, half scan, overscan
___ d. overscan, full scan, half scan

111. Which of the following are used to collimate the primary beam exiting the x-ray tube?

1. pre-patient collimation
2 post-patient collimation
3. beam shaping filters

___ a. 1 and 2
___ b. 1 and 3
___ c. 2 and 3
___ d. 1, 2, & 3

112. What does a pitch of 1.0 represent on a helical or spiral computed tomography unit?

___ a. table increment per 180° equals the section thickness
___ b. table increment per 360° equals the section thickness
___ c. section thickness equals 1 mm
___ d. section thickness equals 1 cm

113. Which of the following problems were acquired by third generation (rotate/rotate) scanners?

    1. detector signal drift sensitivity
    2. spurious signals from moving signal wires
    3. translation motion

    __ a. 1 and 2
    __ b. 1 and 3
    __ c. 2 and 3
    __ d. 1, 2, & 3

114. What is the efficiency range of gas detectors?

    __ a. 1 -5 %
    __ b. 30 - 40%
    __ c. 60 - 90 %
    __ d. 100%

# Image Processing & Display               (#115-130)

115. What is the pixel size if the matrix is 320 x 320 and the field of view is 35 cm?

    __ a. 0.1 mm
    __ b. 1.1 mm
    __ c. 9.1 mm
    __ d. 1,120 cm

116. What units are used to describe the average linear attenuation coefficients acquired by a computed tomography unit?

    __ a. optical density
    __ b. CT or Hounsfield
    __ c. rem or Sv
    __ d. rad or Gy

117. What terms describe the set of pencil thin x-ray beams that strike a detector array?

1. ray
2. projection
3. view

___ a. 1 and 2

___ b. 1 and 3

___ c. 2 and 3

___ d. 1, 2, & 3

118. What change will occur in the number of detected photons if a section thickness is changed from 12 mm to 6 mm?

___ a. decrease 50%

___ b. decrease 25%

___ c. increase 50%

___ d. increase 100%

119. Three-dimensional rendering of contrast media-filled vessels can be obtained by which of the following?

___ a. increasing the display value of contrast media pixels to a maximum density

___ b. drawing a contour line at each contrast media-to-soft tissue interface

___ c. overprojecting contrast media density pixels with adjacent soft tissue pixels

___ d. assigning each pixel with an attenuation coefficient less than the contrast media a value that will display it as transparent

120. What effect does decreasing the field of view have on image display?

___ a. increases image magnification

___ b. decreases image magnification

___ c. increases contrast

___ d. decreases contrast

121. Which of the following is considered a primary advantage to using a filtered back-projection algorithm?

   \_\_ a. calculations can begin after the first profile instead of waiting for the completion of all profiles in a section

   \_\_ b. fewer calculations are necessary for magnified images

   \_\_ c. more calculations permit increased spatial resolution

   \_\_ d. window levels and widths can be preset

122. Which of the following terms defines the conversion of an analog image into numerical data for processing by the computer?

   \_\_ a. scanning

   \_\_ b. sampling

   \_\_ c. digitization

   \_\_ d. quantization

123. An eight-bit ADC (analog-to-digital conversion) will result in how many shades of gray?

   \_\_ a. 2

   \_\_ b. 4

   \_\_ c. 144

   \_\_ d. 256

124. Which of the following terms describes the process of rotating an image by changing the position of the pixels?

   \_\_ a. image enhancement

   \_\_ b. image restoration

   \_\_ c. pattern recognition

   \_\_ d. geometric transformation

125. Which of the following is the most commonly used point processing technique?

   \_\_ a. gray level mapping

   \_\_ b. spatial frequency filtering

   \_\_ c. convolution

   \_\_ d. Fourier domain processing

126. Which of the following describes an image processing operation in which the output image pixel value is determined from a small area of pixels around the corresponding input pixel?

    ___ a. geometric operation

    ___ b. global operation

    ___ c. local operation

    ___ d. point operation

127. Which of the following terms defines a graph of the number of pixels in the entire image or portion of the image plotted as a function of the gray level?

    ___ a. image analysis

    ___ b. histogram

    ___ c. spatial frequency

    ___ d. algorithm

128. Which of the following defines a voxel?

    ___ a. vacillating overscan x-ray exposure limitation

    ___ b. vacuum overload x-ray entrance loading

    ___ c. a system for CT number calculation

    ___ d. volume element

129. Which of the following describes an image processing operation in which the entire input image is used to compute the value of the pixel in the output image?

    ___ a. geometric operation

    ___ b. global operation

    ___ c. local operation

    ___ d. point operation

130. Which of the following lists the three steps of digitization in the correct order?

    ___ a. scanning, sampling, and quantization

    ___ b. sampling, scanning, and quantization

    ___ c. quantization, scanning and sampling

    ___ d. scanning, pattern recognition and sampling

# Image Quality                                      *(#131-141)*

131. Which of the following is true regarding overlapping of sections?

1.  scan time decreases
2.  multiplanar and three dimensional images are smoothed from the extra overlapped data
3.  patient exposure is decreased

    __ a.  1 only
    __ b.  2 only
    __ c.  3 only
    __ d.  1, 2, & 3

132. Which of the following will have an effect on image quality?

1.  spatial resolution
2.  contrast resolution
3.  noise

    __ a.  1 only
    __ b.  2 only
    __ c.  3 only
    __ d.  1, 2, & 3

133. What is the appearance of quantum noise on the computed tomography image?

    __ a.  high contrast
    __ b.  decreased density
    __ c.  poor resolution
    __ d.  grainy

134. Which of the following geometric factors will have an effect on spatial resolution?

1.  focal spot size
2.  detector aperture width
3.  noise

    __ a.  1 only
    __ b.  2 only
    __ c.  1 and 2 only
    __ d.  1, 2, & 3

135. Which of the following terms describes the ability of an imaging system to demonstrate small changes in tissue contrast?

1. low-contrast resolution
2. tissue resolution
3. noise level

___ a. 1 only
___ b. 2 only
___ c. 3 only
___ d. 1 and 2 only

136. Which of the following terms describes the fluctuation of CT numbers from point to point in the image for a scan of uniform material, such as water?

___ a. contrast
___ b. noise
___ c. detector sensitivity
___ d. linearity

137. Which of the following is true regarding aperture size?

___ a. refers to the width of the aperture at the detector
___ b. refers to the width of the aperture at the generator
___ c. refers to the length of the aperture at the multiformat camera
___ d. refers to the length of the aperture at the collimator

138. What are the primary advantages of narrower section thicknesses?

1. improved spatial resolution
2. reduced partial volume averaging
3. higher contrast

___ a. 1 and 2
___ b. 1 and 3
___ c. 2 and 3
___ d. 1, 2, & 3

139. The number of pixels per horizontal and vertical dimensions of the matrix on the monitor screen or film sheet is termed which of the following?

__ a. spatial resolution

__ b. display resolution

__ c. contrast resolution

__ d. high-resolution

140. As section thickness decreases what will happen to the technical factors?

__ a. they will increase

__ b. they will decrease

__ c. they will stay the same

__ d. section thickness has nothing to do with the technical factors

141. Which of the following should be viewed with relatively narrow window widths?

1. orbits
2. mediastinum
3. brain

__ a. 1 and 2

__ b. 1 and 3

__ c. 2 and 3

__ d. 1, 2, & 3

# Artifacts                                    (#142-150)

142. What causes annular ring artifacts typical of third generation scanners?

__ a. one detector out of calibration

__ b. a variety of tissue types within a single voxel

__ c. patient movement

__ d. lack of a proper correction kernel (mathematical filter)

143. What term describes an artifact that may appear on a low dynamic range detector system near the shoulders and hips

because dense bone has too severely attenuated the x-ray beam?

   __ a. beam hardening

   __ b. photon starvation

   __ c. ring

   __ d. partial volume

144. Voluntary and involuntary motion of the patient during CT scanning can result in the appearance of what type of artifact?

   __ a. ring

   __ b. partial volume effect

   __ c. beam restricting

   __ d. streak

145. Which of the following will help to reduce partial volume artifacts?

   __ a. scanning thinner sections

   __ b. scanning thicker sections

   __ c. scanning using a higher technique

   __ d. scanning using a lower technique

146. Which of the following terms defines the increase in the mean energy of a polychromatic beam as it passes through an object?

   __ a. partial volume effect

   __ b. beam hardening

   __ c. cross-field uniformity

   __ d. linearity

147. The term "cupping" artifact can be associated with which of the following terms?

   __ a. motion

   __ b. partial volume effect

   __ c. ring artifacts

   __ d. beam hardening

148. Image artifacts can be created from which of the following?

    1.    motion

    2.    beam hardening

    3.    x-ray tube

    __ a.  1 only

    __ b.  1 & 2 only

    __ c.  2 & 3 only

    __ d.  1, 2 & 3

149. Which of the following artifacts are associated to third generation scanner geometry?

    __ a.  ring

    __ b.  motion

    __ c.  streak

    __ d.  beam hardening

150. Which of the following will produce the most intense motion artifacts?

    1.    arteries

    2.    veins

    3.    stomach gas

    __ a.  1 only

    __ b.  3 only

    __ c.  1 and 2 only

    __ d.  2 and 3 only

# POST-TEST ANSWERS

# Patient Care                          (#1 - 45)

## Patient Preparation                          (#1 - 30)

1. **(B)** The lower portion of the adult sternum is sompressed during CPR. **cardiopulmonary resuscitation (Torres, Adler)**

2. **(B)** Nitroglycerin is a vasodilator used to treat angina pectoris and should be given sublingually (under the tongue). **drugs (Torres, Adler)**

3. **(D)** The intravenous (IV) method of drug administration is selected when the effect of a drug is desired immediately or if a drug cannot be injected into body tissues without damaging them. **intravenous administration (Torres, Adler, Ehrlich)**

4. **(A)** Demeral is a trade name for meperidine hydrochloride, an analgesic with effects similar to morphine. **analgesics (Torres, Adler, Ehrlich)**

5. **(B)** The systolic reading is the highest point reached during contraction of the left ventricle of the heart as it pumps blood into the aorta. **blood pressure (Torres, Adler, Ehrlich)**

6. **(C)** The most important action of a technologist is to prevent the patient from injuring himself during a seizure. **convulsive seizures (Torres, Adler, Ehrlich)**

7. **(D)** A pneumothorax is a collection of air or gas in the pleural cavity. **pneumothroax (Adler, Torres)**

8. **(D)** Ventricular fibrillation is a condition resulting in rapid, tremulous, and ineffectual contractions of the ventricles. If prolonged, this condition can lead to cardiac arrest. **ventricular fibrillation (Adler, Torres)**

9. **(D)** Dyspnea is air hunger resulting in labored or difficult breathing, sometimes accompanied by pain. **dyspnea (Torres, Adler, Ehrlich)**

10. **(C)** Myocardial infarction is a condition caused by an occlusion of one or more of the coronary arteries. The symptoms include prolonged heavy pressure or squeezing pain in the center of the chest behind the sternum. **cardiac failure (Torres, Adler, Ehrlich)**

11. **(D)** Cyanosis is a deficiency of oxygen and excess carbon dioxide in blood caused by gas or any condition interfering with entrance of air into the respiratory tract. **cyanosis (Torres, Adler, Ehrlich)**

12. **(D)** Anaphylatic shock is the form of shock that can result from a severe reaction to a contrast media injection. **shock (Torres, Adler, Ehrlich)**

13. **(A)** Patients will almost all experience a metallic taste following the injection of contrast media. This does not require any type of treatment. **contrast media (Adler, Torres, Ehrlich)**

14. **(B)** Decreasing blood pressure is associated with shock. **medical emergencies (Adler, Torres, Ehrlich)**

15. **(D)** Providing an open airway should be the first priority. **medical emergencies (Adler, Toshiba, Ehrlich)**

16. **(A)** Anaphylactic shock is the type of shock seen most often during CT scanning because it is caused by the use of iodinated contrast materials. **medical emergencies (Torres, Ehrlich)**

17. **(A)** Sodium is the more toxic cation in orgainc ionic contrast media. **contrast media, iodinated contrast agents (Adler, Torres, Ehrlich)**

18. **(B)** Chest-tube drainage systems must always be kept below the chest to allow proper drainage. **chest-tubes (Torres, Adler, Ehrlich)**

19. **(A)** Intussusception is a term that indicates a telescoping of the bowel into itself. **bowel disorders (Haaga, Ballinger, Porth)**

20. **(B)** Portal venous hypertension is a complication of esophageal varices. **esophageal varices (Porth, Haaga, Lee)**

21. **(A)** A transient ischemic attack (TIA) is a sudden cerebral neurologic deficit of presumed vascular origin usually

lasting a few minutes, although they can last up to 24 hours. **medical emergencies (Torres, Adler, Haaga, Porth)**

22. **(A)** A stenosis is a constriction or narrowing of a blood vessel. **stenosis (Torres, Adler, Ehrlich)**

23. **(D)** A diabetic patient whose skin is dry and has a fruity odor on their breath is probably in a diabetic coma. **diabetes mellitus (Torres, Adler, Ehrlich)**

24. **(C)** The most severe form of convulsive seizure is a grand mal seizure. **seizures (Torres, Adler)**

25. **(B)** The desired flow rate and injection time are set and the selected volume in ml/sec will be delivered when using a constant flow rate injector. **automatic injectors (Ballinger, Snopek)**

26. **(A)** A patient should be moved to a lateral recubent or sitting position when vomiting to avoid aspiration of vomitus. **acute emergencies, medical emergencies (Ehrlich, Torres, Adler)**

27. **(C)** Injection time is calculated as volume/time, so $12/2.5 = 4.8$ seconds. **automatic injectors (Ballinger, Snopek)**

28. **(A)** An antihistamine is used to treat (relieve) sympotoms caused by nasal, drug, food, and skin allergies. **contrast adverse reactions (Torres, Adler)**

29. **(A)** The flow rate is defined as the delivery rate or contrast amount delivered per unit of time. **automatic injectors (Snopek, Ballinger)**

30. **(C)** The best CT scan is obtained when scanning is completed before significant interstitial diffusion of contrast media, which occurs within about 2 - 4 minutes after beginning the injection. **drip infusion (Berland, Morgan)**

# Imaging Procedures (#31- #105)

## Head                                                      (#31- #45)

31. **(D)** The sellar floor, suprasellar cistern, and the pititary gland (especially its thickness) would be visualized on a coronal CT scan of the head especiall for examination of the sella. **coronal scans, head, sella (Som, Seeram, Lee)**

32. **(A)** The basil ganglia are gray matter regions of the cerebrum. The caudate nucleus, lentiform nucleus, which is subdivided into the putamen and globus pallidus, and the claustrum make up the basil ganglia. **basil ganglia, cerebrum (Applegate, Akesson)**

33. **(A)** When a hemorrhage has a higher CT number than that of surrounding brain tissue it is considered to be hyperdense. **CT numbers, brain, hemorrhages (Haaga, Som)**

34. **(D)** Spontaneous hemorrhages can occur as a result of hypertensive reactions, rupturing of an aneurysm, and bleeding from an AV malformation. **brain hemorrhages, causes (Haaga, Som, Porth)**

35. **(D)** Direct coronals may be done either supine or prone with the head extended or reformatted coronals may be done from standard head studies. **procedure (Brooker)**

36. **(A)** The inferior nasal concha is illustrated by #1 in Figure PT 1. **CT head, inferior nasal concha, axial imaging (Ellis, Applegate)**

37. **(C)** The maxillary sinus is illustrated by #5 in Figure PT 1. **CT head, maxillary sinus, axial imaging (Ellis, Applegate)**

38. **(B)** The mastoid air cells are illustrated by #3 in Figure PT 1. **CT head, mastoid air cells, axial imaging (Ellis, Applegate)**

39. **(D)** Subdural hematomas are classified as acute, subacute, and chronic. **subdural hematoma, classifications (Haaga, Som, Porth)**

40. **(D)** The scan extent should commence from the beginning of the frontal sinus and proceeds through out the entire sphenoid sinus. Coronal imaging with small sections of 1mm to 3mm are required through the osteomeatal complex. The hard palate is perpendicular to the scan beam. **CT sinuses, procedures (Haaga, Som, Brooker)**

41. **(D)** Taping the head and chin, placing sponges on both sides of the head are meathods of minimizing patient motion. Diazepam (Valium) sedation can only be given with a physicians order. Diazepam injection is not a technologists option. **procedures (Brooker, Seeram, Adler)**

42. **(B)** The angle is 10-20 degrees depending on the area of interest. **procedures (Brooker, Lee)**

43. **(B)** The superior sagittal sinus is illustrated by #1 in Figure PT 2. **CT head, superior sagittal sinus, axial imaging (Ellis, Applegate)**

44. **(A)** The falx cerebri is illustrated by #3 in Figure PT 2. **CT head, falx cerebri, axial imaging (Ellis, Applegate)**

45. **(C)** The thalamus is illustrated by #4 in Figure PT 2. **CT head, Thalamus, axial imaging (Ellis, Applegate)**

# Neck                                                      *(#46-48)*

46. **(A)** CT of the neck requires the patients arms to be placed at the sides of the body and the shoulders should be pulled down as far as possible. **positioning, procedures (Haaga, Lee, Webb)**

47. **(D)** Quiet respiration fills the larynx with air for better definition of the structures. **larynx, procedure (Berland, Brooker)**

48. **(A)** Intravenous contrast media is used differentiate vessels from small nodes and determines a relationship between a mass and blood vessel. Intravenous con-

trast media is not needed to evaluate trauma to the larynx. **contrast media procedures (Haaga, Lee, Webb)**

# Spine                                                    *(#49-59)*

49. **(B)** The most common section orientation that is used for routine scanning of the lumbar spine is the scan orientation is parallel to the intervertebral disc space. **CT lumbar spine, procedures (Haaga, Lee, Webb)**

50. **(C)** The patient's head should be slightly elevated higher than the body following myelography. This will reduce the possibility of post myelography headaches and reduces the possibility of seizures occurring. **CT post-myelography, procedures (Haaga, Lee, Brooker)**

51. **(A)** The most common and recommended scan extent for a routine examination of the lumbar spine is from the mid body of L3 to the top of the sacrum. **CT lumbar spine, scan extent (Webb, Haaga, Lee)**

52. **(A)** It is important that intrathecal contrast media mixes with CSF. By placing the patient in the prone position pooling and layering of contrast media is avoided. **post myelography CT of the spine, intrathecal contrast media (Webb, Lee)**

53. **(C)** Intravenous contrast will enhance scar tissue but not disk. **procedure, spine, contrast (Seeram, Lee)**

54. **(B)** The use of the prone position will decrease the lordosis but would also prevent flexing of the thighs that is done in the supine position. **procedure, spine (Brooker, Haaga)**

55. **(D)** Sacralization of the L5 vertebral body, a rib bearing lumbar vertebrae, and the absence of a lumbar vertebrae are all normal variants that can confuse a technologist when planning the scan extent of an examination of the lumbar spine. **lumbar spine, anatomical variances (Akesson, Webb, Lee)**

56. **(A)** Coronal reformations are useful for determining integrity of spinal fusions and medial and lateral displaced fracture fragments. Sagittal reformations would best demonstrate posteriorly displace fracture fragments

encroaching the spinal canal. **CT spine, multiplanar reformations (Haaga, Lee, Webb)**

57. **(C)** The superior articular process is illustrated by #2 in Figure PT 3. **vertebrae, axial imaging (Ellis, Applegate, Akesson)**

58. **(B)** The inferior articular process is illustrated by #3 in Figure PT 3. **vertebrae, axial imaging (Ellis, Applegate, Akesson)**

59. **(C)** An intervertebral disc space is illustrated by #1 in Figure PT 3. **vertebrae, axial imaging (Ellis, Applegate)**

# Chest *(#60-74)*

60. **(D)** The aorticopulmonary window is a left mediastinal space bounded anteriorly, superiorly, and posteriorly by the ascending aorta, bounded inferiorly by the left pulmonary artery, and bounded medially by the lower trachea and proximal left main bronchus. **CT chest, aorticopulmonary window (Webb, Haaga)**

61. **(D)** It is recommended that dynamic scanning technique at three levels when a dissecting thoracic aneurysm is suspected. **CT chest, dissecting aneurysm, procedures (Haaga, Webb)**

62. **(A)** Image smoothing is reduced because of the use of a bone type algorithm which produces edge enhancement of the interstitial component of the lungs. Spatial resolution is increased and visible image noise is increased. **CT lungs, HRCT (Webb, Seeram)**

63. **(D)** The aortic arch is illustrated by #2 in Figure PT 4. **aortic arch, axial imaging (Haaga, Ellis)**

64. **(A)** The trachea is illustrated by #5 in Figure PT 4. **mediastinum, axial imaging (Lee, Ellis)**

65. **(A)** The superior vena cava is illustrated by #1 in Figure PT 4. **SVC, axial imaging (Ellis, Applegate)**

66. **(A)** HRCT of the lungs requires thin collimation, 1-2mm section thickness would best suit the HRCT technique. **HRCT (Webb, Seeram)**

67. **(D)** Gravity will move fluids to the lowest level and separate densities for better diagnosis. **thorax, preparation, position (Seeram, Brooker, Berland)**

68. **(C)** Suspended expiration provides expansion of the mediastinal structures which provides better visualization of the structures. **respiration, procedures (Lee, Berland)**

69. **(A)** The AP scout view is the most common projection/position obtained. **CT chest, procedures (Brooker, Berland)**

70. **(B)** The right atrium is illustrated by #5 in Figure PT 5. **CT mediastinum, heart (Ellis, Haaga)**

71. **(C)** The descending aorta is illustrated by #3 in Figure PT 5. **CT thorax, aorta (Haaga, Ellis)**

72. **(C)** The left atrium is illustrated by #4 in Figure PT 5. **left atrium, axial imaging (Ellis, Lee)**

73. **(B)** The prone position increases aeration of the posterior lung bases. **thorax, protocols (Seeram)**

74. **(C)** 5mm section thickness combined with 3mm table incrementation provides overlapping scans which will produce the best results when 3D reformation is attempted. **3D reformation, overlap scanning (Seeram)**

# Abdomen                                            (#75-89)

75. **(A)** Scanning prior to the equilibrium phase provides the best opportunity for optimal liver lesion detection. It is important not to start scanning too soon or too late. **CT liver, contrast media injection, procedures (Webb, Haaga)**

76. **(C)** The problem is solved in two steps. First, solve for pitch. Pitch equals table top speed divided by section thickness. 10mm/sec divided by 10mm equals a pitch of 1. Secondly, solve for the total volume scanned. Total volume scanned equals pitch x section thickness x rotations per second x total scan time. 1 x 10 x 1/sec x 30 seconds equals 300mm total volume scanned. **helical/spiral, volume scanning, pitch, total volume (Toshiba, Seeram, Picker, Bushberg)**

77. **(C)** The descending colon is illustrated by #2 in Figure PT 6. **axial imaging, descending colon (Ellis, Applegate)**

78. **(B)** The left renal vein is illustrated by #3 in Figure PT 6. **renal veins, axial imaging (Ellis, Applegate)**

79. **(B)** The left lateral lobe of the liver is illustrated by #1 in Figure PT 6. **CT liver, axial imaging (Ellis, Haaga)**

80. **(B)** 350/WW and 50/WL are adequate for filming soft tissues and 150/WW and 50/WL would provide a "liver window" technique. **windowing, procedures (Webb, Seeram)**

81. **(A)** The smaller the section thickness the better the chance partial volume averaging will not occur, therefore 2mm is the best selection. **partial volume artifacts, section thickness (Berland, Seeram)**

82. **(A)** The use of a low spatial frequency algorithm (standard or smooth) increases low contrast lesion detectability which would be decreased by the use of a high spatial frequency algorithm(bone). **low contrast lesion detectability, low spatial frequency algorithms (Berland, Seeram)**

83. **(D)** All three doses should be given so that the entire GI tract from the stomach to the colon in the pelvis are opacified by contrast. **contrast, procedure, patient (Berland, Brooker, Seeram)**

84. **(C)** An ROI reading of -130 would best demonstrate an attenuation value that is comparable to fat. **CT numbers (Seeram, Adler)**

85. **(B)** Suspended expiration is recommended for abdominal scanning. **respiration, procedures (Berland, Lee)**

86. **(B)** After the ingestion of oral contrast media if the patient is placed in the right lateral decubitus position aids in filling the second portion of the duodenum which would provide an excellent contrast boundary for optimal visualization of the pancreas. **CT pancreas, procedures (Haaga, Lee)**

87. **(B)** A gallstone is illustrated by #4 in figure PT 7. **gallbladder, gallstones (Ellis, Haaga, Lee)**

88. **(C)** The tail of the pancreas is illustrated by #1 in Figure PT 7. **CT pancreas, axial imaging (Ellis, Applegate)**

89. **(C)** The left kidney is illustrated by #2 in Figure PT 7. **kidney, axial imaging (Ellis, Applegate)**

# Pelvis                                                                    *(#90-101)*

90. **(B)** The vas deferens is illustrated by #3 in Figure PT 8. **CT male pelvis, axial imaging (Applegate, Ellis)**

91. **(C)** The urinary bladder is illustrated by #2 in Figure PT 8. **urinary bladder, axial imaging (Ellis, Lee)**

92. **(A)** The rectus abdominis muscle is illustrated by #1 in Figure PT 8. **abdominal musculature, axial imaging (Ellis, Applegate)**

93. **(D)** The uterus, vagina, and the ovaries are all contained within the female true pelvis. **female pelvis, true pelvis (Akesson, Applegate)**

94. **(A)** 500ml of barium sulfate given either introduced rectally just prior to the exam or given orally twelve hours prior to scanning would provide adequate rectosigmoid filling and opacification. **CT pelvis, procedures (Haaga, Lee, Webb)**

95. **(A)** The AP scoutview recommended for CT scanning of the pelvis. **CT pelvis, procedures (Berland, Lee)**

96. **(A)** The percentage of barium in a barium sulfate suspension is 1-3% for abdomen and pelvis computed tomography. **barium sulfate suspension, abdominal CT (Seeram, Lee, Haaga)**

97. **(C)** Contrast within the bladder will help delineate the bladder wall and any associated masses. **preparation, bladder (Berland, Haaga)**

98. **(D)** The levator ani, bulbosponious, and transverse perinei muscles are common in both the male and female pelvis but the orientation of the muscles is different. **pelvic musculature (Applegate, Akesson)**

99. **(C)** The uterus is illustrated by #2 in Figure PT 9. **uterus, axial imaging (Ellis, Haaga)**

100. **(A)** The femoral artery is illustrated by #5 in Figure PT 9. **femoral artery, axial imaging (Ellis, Applegate)**

101. **(C)** The head of the femur is illustrated by #4 in Figure PT 9. **femur, axial imaging (Ellis, Applegate)**

# Musculoskeletal                                    *(#102 - #105 )*

102. **(B)** CT allows better assessment concerning location, orientation, and relationship of fragments in fractures of complex skeletal regions. **musculoskeletal, clinical indications (Seeram)**

103. **(D)** Minimal positioning maneuvers, defining the extent of complicated fractures, and manipulation of acquired data such as windowing techniques and multiplanar reformation makes CT the desired modality for imaging of trauma to the musculoskeletal system. **trauma CT, musculoskeletal system (Haaga, Lee, Seeram)**

104. **(D)** The calcaneus is illustrated by #4 in Figure PT 10. **CT ankle, foot (Ellis, Applegate)**

105. **(A)** The talus is illustrated by #2 in Figure PT 10. **CT ankle, Foot (Ellis, Applegate)**

# Physics and
# Instrumentation *(#106 - #150)*

## System Operation & Components *(#106 - #114)*

106. **(C)** Computed tomography x-ray tubes require anodes capable of handling heavy beat unit loads. Depending on the unit, with 0.5 - 5.0 million heat units may be required. Dynamic and fast scanning units require higher load tube anodes. **computed tomography, x-ray tubes (Carlton, Seeram)**

107. **(D)** Bismuth germanate, calcium fluoride, and gadolinium based ceramic materials are currently being used in scintillation CT detectors. **computed tomography detectors, ionization tubes (Wolbarst, Seeram, Carlton, Bushberg)**

108. **(C)** An array processor increases image processing and display speed by performing simultaneous mathematical operations in a parallel fashion. **digital processing, computer processing, array processor (Carlton, Seeram, Berland)**

109. **(D)** All of the statements are true regarding the highly directional properties of gas filled ionization chamber detectors. This property provides a good acceptance angle for primary x-rays and also assists in rejecting scatter. However, it also eliminates them from use in fourth generation scanners that use a changing alignment between the x-ray beam and detector. **detectors, xenon detectors, gas-filled detectors (Bushberg, Berland, Seeram)**

110. **(A)** A scan arc of 220° is a half scan, a 360° scan arc is a full scan, and a 400° scan arc is an overscan. **scan arcs, half scan, overscan (Berland, Seeram)**

111. **(B)** Pre-patient collimation, fine slit collimation, and beam shaping filters are used to reduce the amount of primary beam reaching the patient, which reduces the amount of secondary scatter produced. Once secondary

scatter has been produced, it is prevented from reaching the detectors by post-patient collimation. **collimation, scatter radiation (Bushberg, Berland, Seeram)**

112. **(B)**  A pitch of 1.0 represent on a helical or spiral computed tomography unit indicates that the table increment per 360° equals the section thickness. **computed tomography: helix, helical, spiral (Bushberg, Seeram)**

113. **(A)**  Detector signal drift sensitivity and spurious signals from moving signal wires were problems that were acquired by third generation scanners. The translation motion was eliminated in the third generation scanners. **computed tomography generation configurations, detectors (Berland, Carlton, Bushberg)**

114. **(C)**  The efficiency range of gas detectors is 60-90%. **computed tomography detectors, ionization chambers (Berland, Carlton)**

# Image Processing & Display          (#115 -130)

115. **(B)**  The pixel size is calculated by dividing the field of view by the matrix size. So, 35 cm/320 = 0.11 cm or 1.1 mm. **matrix, field of view, pixel (Berland, Bushberg, Seeram, Carlton, Hendee)**

116. **(B)**  CT or Hounsfield numbers are the units used to describe the average linear attenuation coefficients acquired by a computed tomography unit. **Hounsfield numbers, CT numbers (Seeram, Bushberg, Berland, Wolbarst, Bushong, Carlton, Curry, Hendee)**

117. **(C)**  The projection or view is the set of rays striking a detector array. The pencil thin x-ray beam that strikes a single detector is referred to as a ray. **projection, view, ray (Bushberg, Berland, Wolbarst, Seeram)**

118. **(A)**  The number of detected photons will decrease by half (decrease 50%) if a section thickness is changed from 12 mm to 6 mm. **section thickness, collimation (Berland, Bushberg, Seeram)**

119. **(D)** Three-dimensional rendering of contrast media-filled vessels can be obtained by assigning each pixel with an attenuation coefficient less than the contrast media a value that will display it as transparent. **three-dimensional display, three-dimensional rendering (Wolbarst, Seeram, Carlton, Bushberg)**

120. **(A)** Decreasing the field of view increases image magnification because each pixel represents less tissue. When the image is displayed with each pixel normal size, anatomical structures appear larger. **magnification, field of view (Carlton, Bushburg, Webb, Seeram, Bushong)**

121. **(A)** A primary advantage to using a filtered-back projection algorithm is that calculations can begin after the first profile instead of waiting for the completion of all profiles in a section. **algorithm, back-projection, Fourier (Wolbarst, Seeram, Bushberg, Carlton)**

122. **(C)** The primary objective when digitizing an image so to convert an analog image into numerical data for processing by the computer, a conversion process known as digitization. **digital processing (Berland, Carlton, Seeram)**

123. **(D)** An eight-bit ADC will result in 256 integers ($2^8$), ranging from 0 to 256, with 256 shades of gray. **digital processing (Berland, Carlton, Seeram)**

124. **(D)** Geometric transformation is a process where images can be rotated or scaled by changing the position of the pixels. **digital processing (Berland, Seeram, Wolbarst)**

125. **(A)** The most commonly used point processing technique is gray level mapping. This is also referred to as contrast enhancement, contrast stretching, histogram modification, histogram stretching, or windowing. **digital processing (Berland, Seeram, Bushong, Wolbarst)**

126. **(C)** A local operation is an image processing operation in which the output image pixel value is determined from a small area of pixels around the corresponding input pixel. These operations are also referred to as area processes or group processes, because a group of pixels is used in the transformation calculation. **digital**

processing (Berland, Seeram, Wolbarst, Bushberg)

127. **(B)**    A histogram is a graph of the number of pixels in the entire image or portion of the image plotted as a function of the gray level. Histograms indicate the overall brightness and contrast of an image. **digital processing (Berland, Seeram)**

128. **(D)**    A voxel is a volume element. **voxel (Seeram, Bushberg, Berland, Wolbarst, Bushong, Carlton, Curry, Hendee)**

129. **(B)**    Global operation is an image processing operation in which the entire input image is used to compute the value of the pixel in the output image. A common example of global operation is Fourier domain processing. **digital processing (Berland, Seeram, Wolbarst)**

130. **(A)**    The primary objective when digitizing an image is to convert an analog image into numerical data for processing by the computer, a conversion process known as digitization. It consists of three distinct steps, scanning, sampling, and quantization. **digital processing (Berland, Seeram, Bushberg, Wolbarst, Kuni)**

# Image Quality                                    *(#131-141)*

131. **(B)**    Multiplanar and three dimensional images are smoothed from the extra overlapped data when sections (sections) are overlapped. **section thickness, overlapping (Berland, Seeram)**

132. **(D)**    Image quality in CT depends on spatial resolution, contrast resolution, noise, and artifacts along with many other factors. **image quality (Berland, Seeram, Carlton, Curry)**

133. **(D)**    Quantum noise appears grainy on the computed tomography image. **noise, section thickness (Berland, Seeram)**

134. **(C)**    Geometric factors refer to factors that play a role in the data acquisition process; these include the focal spot size, detector aperture width, section thickness, distance between the focus, isocenter, detector, and sampling dis-

tance. **image quality (Berland, Seeram, Carlton, Curry, Bushberg)**

135. **(D)** Low-contrast resolution, or tissue resolution, is the ability of an imaging system to demonstrate small changes in tissue contrast. In CT this is sometimes referred to as the sensitivity of the system. **image quality (Berland, Seeram)**

136. **(B)** Noise in CT is the fluctuation of CT numbers from point to point in the image for a scan of uniform material, such as water. **image quality (Berland, Seeram, Carlton, Curry, Bushberg)**

137. **(A)** The aperture size refers to the width of the aperture at the detector. Generally, when the aperture size is smaller than the spacing between objects, the objects can be resolved. **image quality, geometric factors (Berland, Seeram)**

138. **(A)** The primary advantages of narrower section thicknesses are improved spatial resolution in the thickness dimension of the image and reduced partial volume averaging of small objects. Higher contrast is an advantage of wider section thicknesses. **section thickness, acquisition (Bushberg, Seeram, Wolbarst)**

139. **(B)** Display resolution is defined as the number of pixels per horizontal and vertical dimensions of the matrix on the monitor screen or film sheet. Today, CT scanners use higher matrix sizes in conjunction with selected convolution algorithms to improve display resolution. **image quality, reconstruction algorithm (Berland, Seeram, Carlton)**

140. **(A)** As section thickness decreases, the technique factors must be increased. **image quality, contrast resolution (Berland, Seeram, Bushberg)**

141. **(D)** The orbits, mediastinum, and brain are regions of low contrast which require viewing with a relatively narrow window width. **window width (Berland, Seeram, Carlton, Bushong)**

# Artifacts                                            *(#142-150)*

142. **(A)** Annular ring artifacts typical of third generation scanners are caused by one detector being out of calibra-

tion. The further the faulty detector is from the center of the scanning beam, the larger the diameter of the artifact. **artifacts, computed tomography generation configurations (Berland, Bushberg)**

143. **(B)** Photon starvation describes the artifact that may appear on a low dynamic range detector system near the shoulders and hips because dense bone has too severely attenuated the x-ray beam. **artifacts, computed tomography generation configurations (Berland, Bushberg)**

144. **(D)** Motion of the patient during CT scanning can result in the appearance of streak artifacts on the image which appear tangential to the high contrast edges of the moving part. **image quality, image artifacts, motion (Berland, Seeram, Brooker, Bushberg, Wolbarst)**

145. **(A)** Partial volume artifacts appear as bands and streaks. By scanning thinner sections the partial volume artifact can be minimized. **image quality, partial volume effect, image artifacts (Berland, Seeram, Bushberg)**

146. **(B)** Beam hardening refers to the increase in the mean energy of a polychromatic beam as it passes through an object. **image quality, beam hardening, image artifacts (Berland, Seeram, Bushberg, Haaga)**

147. **(D)** A "cupping" artifact can be seen when scanning the brain, and appears as an increase in CT numbers for the soft tissue along the bone-tissue transition of the vault of the cranium. These CT numbers decrease toward the middle of the CT section, hence the term "cupping". This change in CT numbers results in beam hardening artifacts, which appear as broad dark bands or streaks. **image quality, beam hardening, image artifacts (Berland, Seeram, Toshiba)**

148. **(D)** In CT, artifacts arise from a number of sources, including the patient, the CT imaging process itself and the equipment. These artifacts range from those created by motion, metal, and high-contrast sharp edges to those created by beam hardening, partial volume averaging, sampling, detectors, and the x-ray tube. **image quality, image artifacts (Berland, Seeram)**

149. **(A)** Ring artifacts are the result of miscalibration of one detector in a rotate+rotate geometry third generation scanner. **image artifacts, ring artifacts, image quality (Berland, Seeram, Curry, Bushberg, Wolbarst)**

150. **(B)** Motion of objects that have densities much different from their surroundings produce more intense artifacts. Thus, motion of metallic or gas-containing structures produce streaking artifacts. **image quality,. image artifacts, motion artifacts (Berland, Seeram, Curry)**

# Appendix A

# References

Adler, Arlene and Carlton, Richard R. (1994). *Introduction to Radiography and Patient Care*. Philadelphia: W.B. Saunders Publishers.

Akesson, Elizabeth J., Loeb, Jacques A., Wilson-Pauwels. (1990). *Thompson's Core Textbook of Anatomy*. Philadelphia: J.B. Lippincott Company.

Applegate, Edith. (1991) *The Sectional Anatomy Learning System*. Philadelphia: W.B. Saunders Publishers.

Ballinger, P. (1991) *Merrill's Atlas of Radiographic Positions and Procedures*, 7th Edition. St. Louis, MO.: The C.V. Mosby Company.

Behrman, Richard H. Editor. (1994) *Study Guide to Computed Tomography Basic Principles*. Greenwich, Connecticut: Clinical Communications Inc.

Berland, Lincoln L. (1987). *Practical CT Technology and Techniques*. New York: Raven Press.

Brooker, M.J. (1986). *Computed Tomography for Radiographers*. Lancaster: MTP Press Limited.

Bushberg, Jerrold T., Seibert, J. Anthony, Leidholdt, Edwin M., and Boone, John M. (1994). *The Essential Physics of Medical Imaging*. Baltimore: Williams & Wilkins.

Bushong, Stewart. (1993). *Radiologic Science for Technologists,* 5th Edition. St. Louis: CV Mosby Publishers.

Carlton, Richard R. and Adler, Arlene M. (1992). *Principles of Radiographic Imaging*. Albany, NY: Delmar Publishers.

Curry, Thomas S, Dowdey, James E., and Murry, Robert C. (1990). *Christensen's Physics of Diagnostic Radiology,* 4th Edition. Philadelphia: Lea & Febiger.

*Dorland's Medical Dictionary*, 24th Edition. (1989). Philadelphia: W.B. Saunders.

Ehrlich, Ruth Ann, McCloskey Ellen Doble. (1993). *Patient Care in Radiography,* 4th Edition. St.Louis: C.V. Mosby Company.

Ellis, Harold, Logan, Bari, Dixon, Adrian. (1991). *Human Cross-Sectional Anatomy: Atlas of Body Sections and CT Images.* Boston: Butterworth-Heinemann.

Fischbach, Frances Talaska. (1995). *Quick Reference to Common Laboratory and Diagnostic Tests.* Philadelphia: J.B. Lippincott Company.

Haaga, John R. and Alfidi, Ralph J. (1983). *Computed Tomography of the Whole Body, Volumes 1 and 2.* 2nd Edition St.Louis: The C.V. Mosby Co.

Hendee, William R. (1983). *The Physical Principles of Computed Tomography.* Boston: Little, Brown and Company.

Kuni, Christopher C. (1988). *Introduction to Computers and Digital Processing in Medical Imaging.* Chicago: Yearbook.

Lee, Chiu C., Lipcamon, James D., Yiu-Chiu, Victoria. (1994). *Clinical Computed Tomography for the Technologist,* 2nd Edition. New York, New York: Raven Press.

Lee, Joseph K., Sagel, Stuart S., and Stanley, Robert J. (1990). *Computed Body Tomography,* 2nd Edition. New York: Raven Press.

*Mosby's Medical and Nursing Dictionary,* 2nd Edition. (1986). St. Louis: C.V. Mosby.

Noz, Marilyn E. and Maguire, Gerald Q. (1992). *Radiation Protection in the Radiologic and Health Sciences.* 3rd edition. Philadelphia: Lee and Febiger.

Parker, J. Anthony. (1990). *Image Reconstruction in Radiology.* Boca Raton, LA: CRC Press.

Picker International, CT Technical Publications Department. (1993) *Theory of Spiral.* Cleveland, Ohio.

Porth, Carol M., (1994). *Pathophysiology: Concepts of Altered Health States*, 4th Edition. Philadelphia: J.B. Lippincott Company.

Seeram, Euclid, (1994). *Computed Tomography.* Philadelphia: W.B. Saunders Company.

Seeram, Euclid. (1989). *Computers in Diagnostic Radiology.* Springfield, IL: C. Thomas Publishers.

Snopek, A.M. (1992). *Fundamentals of Special Radiographic Procedures*, 3rd Edition. Philadelphia: W.B. Saunders Company.

Som, Peter M., M.D., Bergeron, R. Thomas. (1991) *Head and Neck Imaging,* 2nd Edition. St. Louis: Mosby-Yearbook Inc.

Torres, Lillian S., (1993) *Basic Medical Techniques and Patient Care for Radiologic Technologists,* 4th Edition. Philadelphia: J.B. Lippincott.

Toshiba Corporation, Computed Tomography Department, (1991) *Helical Scanning CT,* Tokyo, Japan: Toshiba Company.

Webb, Richard W., Brandt, William E., Helms, Clyde A., (1991). *Fundamentals of Body CT,* Philadelphia: W.B. Saunders Company.

Wolbarst, Anthony B. (1993). *Physics of Radiology.* Norwalk, CT: Appleton & Lange.

# APPENDIX B

# LABORATORY VALUES

| Test | Standard Value | SI Value |
|---|---|---|
| **Platelet** | | |
| Mosby | 150,000 - 350,000/mm$^3$ | 150 - 350x10$^9$/L |
| Handbook | 150,000 - 450,000mm$^3$ | |
| Stedmans | 150,000 - 350,000/mm$^3$ | 150 - 350x10$^9$/L |
| Miller-Keane | 150,000 - 350,000/mm$^3$ | 150 - 350x10$^9$/L |
| Fischbach | 150,000 - 400,000/mm$^3$ | 150 - 400x10$^9$/L |
| **Blood Urea Nitrogen (BUN)** | | |
| Mosby | 8 - 25mg/100ml | 2.9 - 8.9mmol/L |
| Handbook | 7 - 22mg/dl | |
| Stedmans | 11 - 23 mg/dl | 7.9 - 16.4mmol/L |
| Miller-Keane | 11 - 23mg/dl | 3.9 - 8.2mmol/L |
| Fischbach | 7 - 18mg/dl | 2.5 - 6.4mmol/L |
| **Creatinine** | | |
| Mosby | 15 - 25 mg/kg body weight/d | 0.13 - 0.22mmol kg$^{-1}$/d |
| Handbook | 0.6 - 1.3mg/dl (female) | |
| | 0.8 - 1.5mg/dl (male) | |
| Stedmans | 15 - 25mg/kg body weight/24hr | 0.13 -0.22mmol kg/24hr |
| Miller-Keane | 0.6 - 1.2 mg/dl | 53 - 106 mol/L |
| Fischbach | 0.4-1.5mg/dl | 35 - 132$\mu$mol/L |
| **Prothrombin Time (PT)** | | |
| Mosby | <2 sec deviation from control | <2 sec deviation from control |
| Handbook | 10 - 13sec | 10 - 13sec |
| Stedmans | 12 - 14sec | 12 - 14sec |
| Fischbach | 10 - 14sec | 10 - 14sec |
| **Prothormbin-Plastin Time (Activated) (PTT)** | | |
| Mosby | 25 - 37sec | 25 - 37sec |
| Handbook | 22 - 35sec | 22-25sec |
| Stedmans | 20 - 35sec | 20 - 35 sec |
| Fischbach | 30 - 40sec | 30 - 45sec |

## References

Fischbach, France Talaska. (1995). *Quick Reference to Common Laboratory and Diagnostic Tests*. Philadelphia: J.B. Lippincott Company.

*Handbook of Cardiovascular and Interventioanl Radiography*, Boston: Little, Brown, and Company, 1989.

*Miller-Keane Encyclopedia and Dictionary of Medicine, Nursing, and Allied Health*, 5th Edition, Philadelphia: W.B. Saunders, 1992

Mosby's Medical and Nursing Dictionary, 2nd Edition, St. Louis: C.V. Mosby, 1986.

*Stedmans Concise Medical Dictionary*, 2nd Edition, Baltimore: Williamson and Wilkins, 1994.